THE NATURE OF LAUGHTER

Founded by C. K. Ogden

The International Library of Psychology

GENERAL PSYCHOLOGY
In 38 Volumes

THE NATURE OF LAUGHTER

J C GREGORY

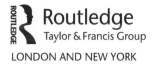

Routledge
Taylor & Francis Group

LONDON AND NEW YORK

First published in 1924 by
Kegan Paul, Trench, Trubner & Co., Ltd.
2 Park Square, Milton Park, Abingdon, Oxfordshire OX14 4RN
711 Third Avenue, New York, NY 10017

First issued in paperback 2014

Routledge is an imprint of the Taylor and Francis Group, an informa business

British Library Cataloguing in Publication Data
A CIP catalogue record for this book
is available from the British Library

The Nature of Laughter
ISBN 978-0415-21022-5
General Psychology: 38 Volumes
ISBN 0415-21129-8
The International Library of Psychology: 204 Volumes
ISBN 0415-19132-7

ISBN 13: 978-1-138-88246-1 (pbk)
ISBN 13: 978-0-415-21022-5 (hbk)

CONTENTS

LAUGHTER

CHAPTER I

SOME VARIETIES OF LAUGHTER

ANGER, like most human emotions, may result in many and diverse actions. An angry man may send his children to bed, cut off his son with a shilling, change his politics, bring a libel suit, write a satire or, reverting to the original and most instinctive manifestation of anger, black his neighbour's eye. This original of all angry methods of attack is apparent in the single action of the animal when impelled by anger : the result of animal rage is usually an assault upon the offender. It is also written upon every human being at the moment of insult. The body of the angered man may be represented by his clenched fist, which is one characteristic expression of his emotion of anger. The extra supply of sugar with which anger floods his blood is typical—as his clenching fist is typical of the pose of his body—of an inward preparation for struggle. Struggle requires energy, and sugar supplies it. The anger diffuses an aggressive poise throughout his whole body, and a preparation for physical attack is evident to the eye in outward manifestation and disclosed to inner physiological exploration. Many other aggressive responses to anger have developed from this original method of physical violence. Anger may be suppressed and it is an important part of moral training to control it, but the single emotion of anger has obviously become connected with many and diverse actions. In anger there is one emotion and many manifestations of it.

On turning from an examination of anger to an inspection of laughter the converse seems to be true. Each member of the row of laughers in Hogarth's picture laughs differently, but every laugh is essentially the same " mechanical motion ", as " dog " is always the same word though written in different hand-writings by twenty different people. This one characteristic bodily action of laughing seems to be connected with many and diverse emotions or feelings. " Emotion " or " feeling " may be intelligibly used to denote the conscious accompaniments of laughter without attempting to conform to accurate definitions of these terms.

As Diomedes stooped to strip his fallen foe of his armour Paris pierced his foot with an arrow. Then Paris leaped to his feet and, " sweetly laughing ", exulted over his enemy.[1]

" Sweetly " seems a strange adjective, for this is the laughter of triumph—laughter in its most crude and brutal form. When Hezekiah desired to unite Israel and Judah in one great passover he made proclamation from Beer-sheba to Dan. " So the posts passed from city to city through the country of Ephraim and Manasseh even unto Zebulun : but they laughed them to scorn " [2]. There is laughter of triumph and laughter of scorn ; there is also laughter of contempt, superiority, and self-congratulation. When lovers laugh as they meet they are not contemptuous, nor are they amused. The pure laughter of play, like the laughter of greeting, is as innocent of amusement as it is of contempt. The ungracious varieties of laughter and the laughter of social delight in greeting and play are often forgotten because human laughter is now so closely associated with amusement. Amused laughter, with its characteristic and indefinable sense of the ludicrous, is a third variety that frequently, in discussions on laughter, draws attention entirely on itself and blinds the mental eye to ungracious forms and laughter of social delight. When the sense of the ludicrous is pure and dispassionately free from either animus or sympathy, amused laughter is purely comic. In humour sympathy blends with the sense of the ludicrous and laughter is transformed from the animosity of triumph or scorn into geniality and friendliness.

Bergson's contrast of humour as scientific satire with the oratorical satire of irony [3] implies another definition for it than a sense of the ludicrous touched with sympathy. But the English tradition favours the distinction between comic laughter whose sympathies are neutral and humorous laughter that is genial and sympathetic. Coleridge distinguished the " pure, unmixed, ludicrous, or laughable " from " the congeniality of humour with pathos " [4] ; " the comic ", wrote Meredith, differs " from satire in not sharply driving into the quivering sensibilities, and from humour in not comforting them and tucking them up " [5], and Professor Saintsbury describes humour " as a feeling and presentation of the ludicrous including sympathetic, or at least meditative, transcendency" [6]. Freud seems to admit the separation of humour from the purely comic through its sympathetic content by suggesting economy of thought as the essence of the latter and economy of *feeling* as the essence of the former [7]. There is authority, therefore, as well as justification through private observation, for distinguishing between the sympathetic laughter of humour and the pure amusement of the comic.

The ungracious, delighted, and amused varieties of laughter do not always, or even usually, occur simple and unmixed. Amusement may mingle with scorn, or contempt with amusement, and social delight may be tinged with triumph. Some writers say that we are deceived by this mingling of emotions into overestimating the number of the varieties of laughter. When Coleridge wrote " to resolve laughter into an expression of contempt is contrary to fact, and laughable enough " [8], he hinted that laughter is never anti-sympathetic and contains no ungracious forms. Mr Max Eastman makes this hint explicit. He urges the dismissal at the outset of scorn and its disagreeable children—including sarcasm, commends Voltaire for affirming the incompatibility of laughter with contempt and indignation, and condemns the first analysts who " confused laughter with the act of scoffing ". Whenever ungracious or unsympathetic elements appear they are pollutions of laughter, not part of it.[9] Thus from the three previous classes of laughter he excludes the first, the ungracious or anti-sympathetic class, leaving the second class of social delight, and the third class of amused laughter. His theory of laughter restricts it to the social delight of greeting or play and the sense of the ludicrous. Professor McDougall restricts further by ignoring all non-amusing forms and defining laughter as " an instinct of aberrant type " that is " accompanied by an emotional excitement of *specific quality*, the quality that is best called ' amusement ' " [10]. This extreme restriction sharply contrasts two possible

5

estimates of laughter. Laughter may have one characteristic emotion, the sense of the ludicrous, and its other varieties may be apparent only because other emotions mingle into its proper emotion. Or it may, as a converse of anger with its single emotion and many actions, have one action of body and many, perhaps very many, emotions.

Any advance in knowledge can, from one point of view, be described as a progressive disclosure under scrutiny, as a white patch far distant up the road divides, as it approaches the observer, into a flock of sheep and as each member of the flock, on nearer approach or on closer observation, reveals its value as wool or mutton. There has been much thinking and much writing on laughter, but its progressive disclosure of itself to scrutiny has been, admittedly, very small. This reluctance of laughter to disclose its own nature increases the importance of holding firmly to what can be known. The decision between singleness and multiplicity in laughter which study meets at the outset cannot be dogmatically or assuredly made. But, since it does seem possible to discover some elements in laughter, though they may be few, that favour its multiple nature, it seems to be wise method to assume at the beginning a connection between the act of laughing and a variety of emotions. As the argument proceeds on this preliminary assumption it will be found to include still more kinds of laughter than have been already described. These further varieties of laughter seem to be as clearly different species as those included in the three classes so ruthlessly reduced to one single kind by Professor McDougall. If there are many ways of laughing these seemingly additional species are of them. If the final decision falls on singleness for laughter they will be condemned as false appearances along with all ungracious laughing and even, if Professor McDougall has his way, along with the laughter of greeting or of play. Congruency with the facts of laughter, so far as these can be discovered, must ultimately decide between the rival hypotheses. If the monistic view of laughter, as McDougall's theory may be conveniently called, most adequately coordinates the facts and estimates of them, it will prevail. If Eastman's concession of one or two extra varieties to laughter co-ordinates most adequately, his modestly pluralistic theory will prevail over McDougall's. If the freely pluralistic estimate, as it may be called to contrast it with the monistic, is more adequate than the other two, it will prevail over them both. It will be assumed here that there are many laughters : laughters of triumph, of scorn and contempt, of superiority, of self-congratulation, of play, of greeting, and of amusement, which includes pure comic perception of the ludicrous and

7

humour with sympathy. Other varieties will be involved in the connection of these with the fundamental facts of laughter. The following chapters will present laughter in terms of the hypothesis that it has had, and still has, many varieties. No dogmatism is intended, for laughter eludes all dogmatism and laughs at it, but an attempt is simply made to identify some features of human laughter and to connect them consistently.

CHAPTER II

THE traditional sourness of the dwarf, or misshapen person, is, when properly understood, an index of the humanization of laughter. Since men suit their conduct to their treatment, habitual ridicule breeds temper in the ridiculed, and the dwarf of tradition was bitter because he was an object of merriment. The passing of this tradition, as sympathy replaces derision, marks a humanization in the occasions of men's laughter.

The lives of Sir Francis Bacon, Thomas Fuller, and Thomas Hobbes covered the 118 years from 1561 to 1679, and these three writers thus represent the thought and habit of a period from 250 to 300 years before the present. They all revealed the mind of their times by recording the objects of men's laughter. "Deformity" heads Bacon's list [11], and "infirmities" are emphasized by Hobbes [12]. "Infirmity" is used more widely than in a purely physical sense by Hobbes, but Fuller's protest against beating "a cripple with his own crutches " or mocking " a cobbler for his black thumbs ", in his chapter " Of Jesting ", implies that physical infirmities were, in that age, recognized objects of mirth[13]. England in the seventeenth century simply continued a cruel habit of making merry over physical misfortunes. When the Philistine lords made sport of blind Samson[14] they were mocking an enemy, and revenge always stirs bitterness, but the glee of Olympus over the limping Hephæstus, as he bustled through the palace[15], doubtless represents the spirit in the laughter of the time, as Bacon, Fuller, and Hobbes represent the spirit of theirs. This glee over physical infirmity is too evident in a survey of the past that reviews the occasions of men's laughter for these instances not to be typical. Human mirth has always been easily aroused by the spectacle of physical infirmities.

There is still such mirth, but, since deformity is no longer a legitimate object of laughter and among the highly civilized no longer provokes it, it is clear that laughter has been humanized. The growth of the sympathetic spirit has affected laughter, and, if there is an index to the progress of civilization, the degrees of failure in sympathy discovered when men laugh may provide it. The disappearance of physical infirmity as a recognized object of mirth intimates a wider spread and a deeper planting of the spirit of sympathy. Man has become more humanized : his sympathies have moved with his civilization and his laughter has moved with both.

Ungraciousness and spite have been too prevalent and too persistent in laughter to be only pollutions of it. A survey of the occasions of laughter in the past suggests that men never have laughed and never will except at some form of humiliation. Though highly civilized men may no longer laugh at some misfortunes, such as physical infirmity, they seem to some who have made this survey only to have restricted the anti-sympathetic elements in their laughter without any positive introduction of sympathy. It is possible to over-emphasize that the ancients " were impressed with the sane and wholesome humour of superiority " [16]. The Greek warriors " laughed lightly " when Thersites bowed and wept under the staff of Odysseus, for they were pleased that a prater had been silenced. But Homer hints at humanization by adding " though they were sorry " [17]. Nor must we forget that Plato would not permit ridicule of citizens, even without anger [18]. But malignity, contempt, and the stroke of superiority pervaded ancient laughter. When Socrates cited the impotent as natural objects of laughter his citation was more incidental than the deliberate citations of Bacon and Hobbes, and when he mentioned pleasant laughter, made tart by envy, at the follies of friends, he was not analysing mirth [19]. But his selection of occasions for laughter is significant. Plato clearly considered laughter to be an inferior thing, for, though the serious man must understand laughable things if he would understand serious matters, he should leave the ridiculous to slaves and hired strangers [20], and jests " which you would be ashamed to make yourself " touch " a principle within which is disposed to raise a laugh " [21]. He feared immoderate laughter in the guardians of his State and would suffer no Homeric description of laughter among the blessed gods as they watched the bustling Hephæstus [22]. Glee among gods over deformity shocked Plato, and doubtless the frequent cruelty and constant hardness in ancient laughter determined his disparagement of comedy and the ludicrous. Thus Plato's depreciation of laughter is a witness to its constant ungraciousness in the pre-Christian world and all amusement seemed to him to be too hard for penetration by human sympathy.

Since Mr Lloyd speaks of the " humour of superiority " and thinks the humorist can always appeal safely to this sentiment [16], he may have a similar opinion about the laughter of the Christian world. Perhaps, for there is no exact science of laughter and no accepted precision in terms, he merely does not assign the name " humour " exclusively to sympathetic laughter. He rightly recognizes the persistence of the aggressive element in the pervasive sense of the ludicrous—which he always calls " humour." The smiting of Thersites, the limping of Hephæstus, and the comedy of Aristophanes doubtless do appeal to the sense of physical superiority which survives in the " humour " of competitive races. Lashing imposture and exposing hypocrisy no doubt still appeal to the French. The exposure of dignity in *déshabillé*, it may be added, or the shattering of pretensions, by ridicule, is still sure of a laugh.

As laughter emerges with man from the mists of antiquity it seems to hold a dagger in its hand. There is enough brutal triumph, enough contempt, and enough striking down from superiority in the records of antiquity and in its estimates of laughter to presume that original laughter may have been wholly animosity. If this were so, as will appear in the sequel, it probably contained from the first, at least, the germ of future kindliness. But there is an unquestionable brutality in the ancestry of laughter. It is tempting to discover a survival of this original brutality in the publics, the audiences collected at popular entertainments, of western civilizations. Mr Max Beerbohm may be too unsympathetic towards crowds to be perfectly discerning when he finds " two elements in the public's humour : delight in suffering,

contempt for the unfamiliar " [23]. Socrates
once stood up when Aristophanes represented
him on the stage and Mr Eastman's remark
that Athenian humour was probably more
exuberant than hostile [24] may carry a
correction of the Beerbohm opinion. Though
crowds, like individuals, constantly incline to
laugh derisively, they should probably be
credited with more sympathetic laughter
than Mr Max Beerbohm allows to them.

Children, who hint at the history of their
race without repeating it precisely, seem to
disclose the original and persistent unkindness in laughter. If Mr Beerbohm is rightly
suspected of injustice to publics, he may also
be suspected of injustice to children : it is
natural, he says, for the unsophisticated
public to laugh gleefully at suffering and
contemptuously at the unfamiliar, because it
will laugh as children laugh [23]. Nor, even
though children are convicted of deficiency
in a sense of the comic, is their laughter
necessarily convicted of delight in suffering. Freud [25] thinks they do lack feeling for
the comic, and Mr St John Lucas agrees with
him, though mainly, apparently, because he
was a serious boy himself [26]. But, though
children are unkind laughers neither because
an essayist says they are nor because their
laughter must be unkind since it has little
sense of the ludicrous, statistical inquiry seems
to be against them. Dr Kimmins noted the

element of superiority in " children's sense of humour " and at nine years old a pleasure in ridicule of the school-inspector. It is perhaps significant that when the child's appreciation of the comic falls off from eleven to thirteen, after increasing up to eleven, the element of superiority is exaggerated[27]. The appearance of unkindness as laughter begins, and as appreciation of the comic temporarily wanes, suggests the primacy of scorn and contempt in human mirth.

The hint in the laughter of the child, and perhaps in the laughter of the crowd, that unsympathetic or anti-sympathetic laughter preceded the humorous is realized in history. Laughter has steadily become, though with many a fluctuation, more gracious, genial, and kindly. This steady tendency towards humour from less gracious forms is reflected in a contrast between the older and some of the modern theories of laughter. A sense of the humanization of laughter, of its modern growth towards the humorous, is apparent in this contrast. Since a full survey of theories of laughter would be tedious if not impossible, a representative of the old must be chosen to contrast with a representative of the new. Whether their theories are right or wrong, these two representatives will be found, in one point of contrast between their estimates of laughter, to intimate a sense that laughter has been humanized.

The choice of the first representative falls almost inevitably on Thomas Hobbes. His definition of laughter is one of the most famous in the history of thought, and he sufficiently represents the anti-sympathetic estimate of laughter, once almost universal and still widely held, to point a contrast with the modern sympathetic estimate. The " sudden glory " with which he identified the " passion of laughter " felicitously expresses the warm flush of emotion as laughter floods the soul. It arises from a " sudden conception of some eminency in ourselves " : identifying laughter with self-congratulatory superiority. It is born in unkindness, for this sense of eminency comes " by comparison with the infirmities of others ". Hobbes almost stirs us to compunction at choosing him to represent derision theories by immediately adding that " men laugh at the follies of *themselves* past, when they come suddenly to remembrance, except they bring with them any present dishonour " He also contemplates non-derisive laughter when he thinks laughter may be " without offence " if it is " at the absurdities and infirmities *abstracted from persons* " [28]. Many writers have estimated laughter as more essentially derisive than Hobbes. But he can be spokesman for anti-sympathetic theories, though he attributes less vindictiveness to the laugh than many of the many whom he represents. " The many " can be used very advisedly, for an anti-sympathetic estimate of laughter was widespread both before and after he wrote. It persists still : intimidation by humiliation is for Bergson the function of laughter [29]. However the theory of Hobbes is described, as " derision ", which is doubtfully just, as " superiority " or " self-congratulatory ", it depends laughter upon unsympathetic or anti-sympathetic impulses.

Hobbes emphasized the structure or mechanism of laughter ; modern theories emphasize its function. He told us what laughter is ; Professor McDougall tells us what laughter does. But this difference of emphasis does not conceal another significant contrast. According to Hobbes men laugh when they have too little sympathy ; according to McDougall they laugh to avoid having too much. Sympathy tends to become too sensitive, and if it is not corrected minor mishaps would stir men too easily. So, when a member of the old Parliament sat down on his hat, his fellow-members laughed instead of condoled. " Minor " mishaps may be minor absolutely or minor relatively. They may be too inconsiderable to need sympathy, or too remote from the observer in time, space, and circumstance to secure it. Sometimes the mishap ought not to receive sympathy : the ruffling of senatorial dignity may be good physic. When wit exposes folly laughter may be a better medicine than condolence. Thus

" laughter is primarily and fundamentally the antidote of sympathetic pain", and its " biological function " is " defence of the organism against the many minor pains to which man is exposed by reason of the high sensitivity of his primitive sympathetic tendencies." [30]

If laughter has been progressively humanized, it is natural to discover a keener sense of the connection between laughter and sympathy in the recent than in the older writer. McDougall notes that we can laugh at " our dearest friend " and simultaneously " sincerely condole with him ". The difference between Hobbes, who thought that we laugh because we are not sympathetic, and McDougall, who thinks that we laugh because we incline to sympathize too much, marks a sense of the humanization of laughter. A modern writer like Eastman is amusing in his perplexity over Hobbes and his followers. He cannot understand unsympathetic or anti-sympathetic theories. There need be no perplexity if Hobbes lived in a less sympathetic age than the present. Laughter has responded to the growth of sympathy and become more sympathetic itself. A survey of laughter and a comparison of estimates of its nature show that it has steadily tended to become less contemptuous and more sympathetic. If we arrange laughters in a series, from triumph or scorn to a sympathetic sense of the ludicrous, that series represents a steady humanization into humour, which is the constant goal of civilization and the final achievement of laughter.

If there are many laughters and if there has been evolution among them they probably contain a fundamental element. The ground-plan of laughter, the primary situation in which laughter always arises, does not seem to be far to seek. Most theories of laughter have recognized it in some form, though its full significance is not always appreciated. There is an element in all laughter that seems obvious, productive of its varieties and naturally connected with its growth in sympathy. It does not remove all enigmas from laughter, nor complete explanation, but it does make laughter partly intelligible. This element needs no great analytical skill to expose it nor arduous reflection to perceive it, for it is simply the familiar, and even obtrusive, element of *relief*.

CHAPTER III

ABOUT fifty years ago two companion prints hung in many houses on opposite walls or cheek by jowl. They were long and narrow, and each represented a row of children in school. The dux sat at one end and the dunce, wearing the traditional cap, stood on a stool at the other. The remaining scholars sat between them, presumably in the order of what would now be called their coefficients of intelligence. In one picture the children bent seriously over their task—even the dunce kept his eyes on his book. Underneath this picture was printed " The Frown ". In the companion-picture the same row of children, from dux to dunce, sat, or stood, cheerfully and at ease. Underneath this picture was printed " The Smile ". A single glance at the two prints appreciated a fundamental element in laughter. The observer *felt* the change from those tense, studious bodies to these cheerful, relaxed urchins, and experienced, almost as if he sat in the smiling row, the burst of *relief* as the teacher smiled.

Laughter has been so pervaded by a sense of the ludicrous that sheer unsophisticated laughter of pure relief is seldom untinged by amusement. Washington Irving was wakened on Christmas morning by little voices singing carols outside his chamber-door. When he looked out the little group of children became mute, and each child shyly hung its head. Then, of one accord, they scampered down the corridor and Irving heard them laughing as they turned the corner [31]. This little incident almost catches the sense of the ludicrous in the act of birth from a situation of relief, for the children laughed first because their fears had relaxed and only secondarily because they were amused. In the evolution of laughter—so this little incident prompts us to surmise — amusement has insinuated itself into situations of relief. It began with mild insinuation, so the surmise runs, and has ended by taking over laughter as its special province. But the dominance of laughter by the sense of the ludicrous is not complete enough to obliterate either the many laughters into which amusement merely mingles or those into which it does not enter at all.

To the ungracious laughters from triumph to mild superiority, the laughters of greeting and of play and laughter at the ludicrous, which may be purely comic or sympathetically

humorous, must be added the sheer laughter
of relief. "At the sacrificial altar, during the
Roman festival of the Lupercalia, two young
men would be touched with a bloody knife,
and, when the blood had been wiped from
their foreheads with a handful of wool dipped
in milk, the ritual required that they should
laugh" [32]. This was, doubtless, a dwindled
ritual relic of a sacrifice in which the " two
young men ", or the victims they represented,
were actually slain. Since the comic has no
place in the solemnity of sacrificial ritual,
laughter was estimated, and ritualistically
required, as an expression of relief. Laughter
was *estimated*, it should be noted, as relief,
or as an index of it. " I couldn't help but
laugh ", said a spectator of the anguish of
women who were seeking news of shipwrecked
men at a London dock, and soldiers have
laughed " when a shell took off a comrade's
hand " [33]. The sheer relief of such events,
whether in the participator who escapes in
person or in the observer who watches a peril
that passes him touch others, marks a distinct
species of laughter. Often, when laughter is
less sheerly pure relief, a situation of relief is
clearly its origin. The soliloquizer in the
churchyard, " reading the various inscriptions,
and moralizing on them with that kind of
levity, which will not infrequently spring up
in the mind, and in the midst of deep melancholy ", wondered jestingly " where be all the

bad people buried " [34]. The jest often appears as an interloper in the midst of seriousness when the tension temporarily falls and then announces its own birth from a relaxation of the spirit. The passing of crisis prepares a path for laughter : during the annular eclipse of October 1919 the Gold Coast natives fled trembling to their huts ; when it was over they laughed at their own fears [35]. These transitions from relief to amusement, where the transition is obvious enough to suggest the genesis of the sense of the ludicrous, hint at an original laughter of pure relief. A woman who was caught in machinery and just saved from mutilation or death, threw herself on a table and laughed. She laughed from impulse and the discharged Lupercalian victims laughed by instruction, which perhaps also touched an impulse to laugh from relief and was doubtless based on it, but they all laughed for the same reason. That reason was liberation from danger, and a sheer sense of relief is one clearly distinguishable, and perhaps the most fundamental, emotional accompaniment of laughter.

Relief is written legibly on many varieties of laughter : on triumph, with its exultant pause after consummated struggle ; on scorn, which contains contempt for a futile menace ; on superiority with its easy assurance that its victim is no serious rival. It is written, though perhaps less legibly, on the laughter of greeting. Two human beings cannot meet neutrally, for each calls upon the other to meet a social situation. In prehistoric days, and perhaps long after, there was always a possible menace in a meeting, and a subdued menace is still present in a doubtfulness over the conduct required for the interview. A preparedness for eventualities, a hesitancy about the character of the interviewed, a constraint naturally arising from uncertainty, suffuse the interviewer. When friend meets friend the social tension rises only to fall and relief passes quickly into laughter or smiling : friends, according to Penjon [36], experience an increase of liberty when they meet. The more formal greetings between strangers intimate uncertainty about one another and contrast with the greater familiarity between friends. The laughter of greeting is part of this familiarity, which, like all familiarity, decreases constraint. The relief in the laughter of play is written all over children as they escape from school.

Relief is too unmistakable in most laughter that is free from amusement or only tinged by it to be unobserved. It is evident also in a survey of the comic and the humorous. A workman engaged in blasting operations dallied too long and went up with the charge. As the unfortunate man went upwards, the foreman drew out his notebook. When the workman received his week's pay a sum corresponding to the time he had spent in the air was deducted from his wage. The beginning of this story makes a big call on sympathy and the end makes a small one. It is distressing to have even sixpence deducted from one's wage, but it is much more distressing to be dashed into pieces. The sympathies rapidly collected for the major distress are suddenly required only for the minor, and relief clearly pervades the laughter that greets the story.

A survey of the occasions of laughter discovers always, sometimes clearly, sometimes less distinctly and sometimes, perhaps, with difficulty, but discovers always, the common element of relief.

The relief written on all varieties of laughter is also written on its " peculiar bodily reactions ". Descriptions of the mechanics of laughter vary from snatch-phrases, through effective portraiture, to systematic and accurate analysis. The " distortion of the countenance ", like the bush that denoted a wine-shop, is no more than an obvious " sign " of laughter, nor did Hobbes intend a physiological study[37]. Bacon draws a more careful picture : " laughing causeth a dilatation of the mouth and lips ; a continued expulsion of the breath, with a loud noise, which maketh the interjection of laughing ; shaking of the breasts and sides ; running of the eyes with water, if it be violent and continued "[38]. Leigh Hunt[39] particularly

25

describes how " the breath recedes only to reissue with double force " and summarizes the rest as a " happy convulsion ". The details, of this " happy convulsion ", as Bacon supplies them and as Darwin has carefully studied them [40], can be ignored in favour of the " continued expulsion of the breath ", the rapid succession of breathing in and breathing out that indicates the essential significance of the mechanics of laughter. Sully [41] emphasizes the deepening of inspiration and breaking up of expiration. If laughter is regarded as an enhanced giggle or magnified titter, to which it constantly descends, its significance is plain. We hold our breath, or draw it in, to prepare for effort ; when we abandon effort we let our breath out. The titter or giggle draws and lets with constant alternation, and the laugh does the same more vigorously. A sudden call for effort and a sudden call off are repeated in rapid alternation during the explosions of laughing. Now this is simply a periodic expression of relief : a call upon effort being apparent as " the breath recedes " and a call off in its " reissue with double force ". Milton's " laughter holding both his sides " expresses in terse, palpable summary the relieved effort of laughter [42].

An Irishman might say of laughter that it does something without doing anything. The body prepares for action and then, since effort is cut short, expends its preparation on itself :

26

" the happy convulsion " is a spill-way for gathered energy, as Herbert Spencer perceived[43]. This expenditure of summoned energy upon itself by the convulsed body, which is more external in visible " mechanical motion ", seems to extend through the whole organism. Every call upon the body for action prepares it internally for effort by " energizing secretions." Anger, which poises the body for a blow and prepares it internally for struggle, is typical of any call for action, and the extra sugar that it stimulates into the blood is typical of all such internal preparation. The call for action with which the situation resulting in laughter begins increases the sugar in the blood. This sugar, and the other associated secretions, supply an extra source of energy. When action is called off this extra store of energy producers would remain in the body and become, since unrequired, waste products. These waste products would clog the body, which would be like a fire with too much fuel. Laughter, therefore, Dr Crile suggests, substitutes for action *by* the body action *of* or *in* the body and thus consumes the " energizing secretions "[44]. This substitutionary role of laughter explains the somewhat puzzling repetitiveness in laughing. An action has been prepared for and an action must occur if waste products are not to clog the body, so laughter continually rehearses the situation of calling on and calling off to provide a physical exercise that will use up the sugar and its associates. If laughter is such a transference from an external to an internal gymnastic and, physiologically, a clearance of unnecessary substances, it is as obviously determined by relief in this aspect as it is in its aspect of respiration. Relaxation by interrupted effort is written on the repetitive interruption of inspiration and on the sweeping away of sugar which is no longer needed.

Thus laughter is an action diverted from its original intention of affecting persons or things outside the body and directed exclusively upon the body itself. It responds to a call for action that is quickly called off, and expends a preparation for effort upon the body because it has become otherwise useless. The *relief* thus immanent in the act of laughing stands out sharply when contrasted with the act of crying. Crying, like laughing, " is primarily an act of the respiratory muscles " [45] : sobbing may be summarily described as sorrowful tittering or a giggle as a glad sob. An action called on and then called off is apparent in the spasmodic breathing of both. But, in crying, action is called off because it is futile, and in laughter because it is not needed. Thus, though the two are akin and, as has often been noted, pass readily into one another, crying is sorrowful because endeavour is vain and laughter is joyful because effort is relaxed. In its visible aspect, in its physiological function, and in its contrast with weeping, laughter is plainly and obviously an expression of *relief*.

Relief is the constitutive element in the physical act of laughing : laughter, physiologically, releases the body from a necessity for exertion and relieves it of secretions. The characteristic emotion of one variety of laughter seems to be a pure sense of relief. In many other varieties relief is too obvious in the associated emotions to be mistaken. When it is less obvious it can still be observed. An element so pervasive of laughter, so deeply penetrative into many of its varieties and so characteristic of its physical expression, can hardly be other than the common, fundamental ground-plan of all laughters, the centre or source from which they all spring.

The relief characteristic of laughter is not a long period of ease but a sharp withdrawal of a demand. " Merriment ", wrote Dr Johnson, " is always the effect of a sudden impression " [46], and it would be tedious to catalogue the insistences of eminent writers, from the " sudden glory " of Hobbes till now, upon the suddenness in laughter. In laughter there is a *psychical shock*, which Dr Johnson discerned in " the pleasures of the mind ". All mental pleasures, he said, " imply something sudden and unexpected ", and it is certainly true of the delight derived from a sense of the ludicrous that " what is perceived by slow

29

degrees . . . will never strike with the sense of pleasure " [47]. A joke may dawn upon the mind, but laughter ensues at the decisive moment of perception when obtuseness is sharply succeeded by insight. The satisfaction of sheer relief is sudden, and triumph bursts into laughter with the stroke of success. Suddenness pervades all laughter, for it is an essential element in its fundamental quality of relief.

The members of the world of life do not develop into one another in single file : they occur in groups springing from common centres and not in one simple series like the numbers 1 to 100. Differently specializing animals develop out of a generalized type [48]. The primitive four-limbed animal had mobile, propellent limbs. An ordinary water-newt, clambering over obstacles at the bottom of its tank or climbing up aquatic plants, approximates to and represents, though it is not identical with, the central generalized form from which the variously specializing four-limbed animals developed. The horse has converted each limb into a stable prop and an aid to swift movement : it has sacrificed all other advantages to standing, walking, or running. Some monkeys, instead of acquiring four legs, have acquired four arms with hands. Man has two legs and two hands. The horse sacrificed mobility, or reaching, stretching, and grasping power, to stability ;

the four-handed monkeys kept all their limbs mobile and man has reserved two limbs for stability and two for mobility. From a leg-less and handless ancestor, with four poten-tial legs or arms ending in hands, different animals developed which specialized differently in realizing the primitive potentiality. The horse, four-handed monkeys, and man are only three lines of development out of many that radiated from the original centre. The completeness of specialization into leg and arm and the mode of distributing functions among all four limbs varied from group to group of specializing animals[49]. This radia-tion in lines of growth from an original source is constantly repeated in the world of life. The appearance presented by a flight of shooting stars is a natural diagram of this constantly repeated plan of growth. All the stars in one flight appear to stream from one radiant point, and animals and plants constantly do in reality what the stars, which actually move in parallel paths, seem to the eye to do.

The varieties of laughter probably conform with this plan, with relief as their common source. Triumphant laughter need not be the lineal ancestor of humour, though both have a common origin. A directness of ancestry between the laughters of triumph and humour was implied by George Eliot : " Strange as the genealogy may sound, the original parentage of that wonderful and delicious mixture of fun, fancy, philosophy, and feeling which constitutes modern humour was probably the cruel mockery of a savage at the writhings of a suffering enemy " [50]. The " genealogy " need not be rejected because it is " strange ", for it is characteristic of all life to grow away from its source. An oak very successfully conceals its birth from an acorn—who, if he were shown an oak and an acorn for the first time and were ignorant of the growth of plants, would believe they were parent and child ? The brutality in crude, barbarous laughter of battle-triumph could soften into the sympathy of humour, though the laughters of triumph, scorn, and other ungracious forms may not stand in a simple step-by-step series with the laughters containing a sense of the ludicrous. For, however the relationship between brutal and sympathetic laughters is conceived, whether as linear or radiate from a centre, there is an obvious connection between the humanization historically evident in laughter and the fundamental element of relief. Laughter has been responsive to the growth of human sympathy, and it has been responsive because its relief has enabled it to respond.

Triumphant laughter is exultant because the foe is beaten and no further stroke is needed. Scornful laughter feels safe in the presence of an impotent threat. Assured victory or the certainty of it if a despised

threat passes into action prompts to a contemptuous mercy. Since laughter, when it
springs from triumph, is a blow cut short, a
stroke diverted from an enemy and expended
pleasantly upon self, it tends, as Sydney
Smith remarked, to diminish hatred, as per-
spiration diminishes heat [51]. Anger and all
aggressive emotions appear in the human
being tense for action and remain till the
final stroke is made ; they perish naturally
in the relief of laughter when there is no need
to strike and aggression is at an end. The
ending of aggression, which is a necessary consequence of laugher, does not necessarily
purge the laughter of all hostility nor result
in prompt sympathy. But it obviously provides an opportunity for sympathy to enter.
The contemptuous mercy of the exultant and
laughing conqueror is not the rich sympathy
of humour, but it is an earnest of the possibility inherent in the nature of laughter that
has been realized in its humanization. Relief,
by cutting short the hostile act and breaking
in upon the hostile mood, is a step towards
sympathy. According to the Sāṃkhya
system of Indian philosophy we secure results
by removing obstacles, as we fill a bath by
turning a tap [52]. Animus is the constant
obstacle to sympathy, and the relief of
laughter tends to remove it. Sympathy, as
its progressive humanization of laughter reveals, has constantly flowed in through the

interruption of animus by relief until the "humorous writer", in the words of Thackeray, "professes to awaken and direct your love, your pity, your kindness—your scorn for untruth, pretension, imposture—your tenderness for the weak, the poor, the oppressed, the unhappy" [53].

Paradoxically, animus lingers in the laugh for the same reason that it leaves it. Most writers appreciate this persistent clinging of relics of animus to laughter. The more brutal laughters, though they exist yet, have receded before the more sympathetic, but laughter is still, as it may always be, a gratification of the sense of superiority and an effective social discipline. This double tendency in laughter to extend and withdraw sympathy is described by Sydney Smith in two nearly successive estimates : laughter reduces hatred but "the object of laughter is always inferior to us" and the sense of the humorous is incompatible with tenderness and respect [54]. Thackeray interpolates "scorn for untruth, pretension, imposture" between the love, pity, and kindness aroused by "the humorous writer" and the "tenderness for the weak, the poor, the oppressed, the unhappy" he promotes : animus creeps in and out of laughter to suit the occasion. Sydney Smith, if his estimates of humour are collated, seems to think of it as restricted animus. "Incongruities which excite laughter generally produce a feeling of

contempt for the person at whom we laugh " :
there is always some animus in amusement.
But violent animus ruins laughter : " contempt verges on anger, and the humorous is
at an end " [55]. A sense of this restricted
animus appears in Bain's opinion of " a sudden
stroke of superiority " as one of the most
certain " causes of the outburst of laughter " [56]
and continues, with the degree of restriction
more or less severely estimated, in many
modern theories of laughter. Less leniently,
Bergson establishes a somewhat higher degree
of animus in laughter by dubbing it " social
ragging " and convicting it of " an unavowed
intention to humiliate " [57].

The restricted animus of laughter, according
to Bergson, is applied as social discipline to
punish human beings for acting like machines,
or automata, instead of meeting circumstance
with plasticity and initiative, as living beings
should. The laughable element is " mechanical inelasticity " ; absent-mindedness and
eccentricity are restrained by the " social
gesture " called laughter ; human actions are
ludicrous in an exact proportion to their
simulation of machinery. Imitation is amusing, and two like faces are ludicrous because
both suggest a manufacturing process. Cere-
monial has a latent comic element ; Jack-in-
the-Box and Punch and Judy arouse laughter
because puppets pretend to be living ; " the
ludicrous in events may be defined as absent-

mindedness in things ". Inadvertence is one main source of the comic, and parody, degradation, exaggeration, unsociability provoke laughter, which always " indicates a slight revolt on the surface of social life " and intimidates by humiliation [58]. Bergson selects one obvious function of laughter to make it sole and exclusive. Eccentricity reigns in Bedlam, Sydney Smith noted, because the eccentrics are undeterred by each other's laughter [59]. Few would dissent from the dictum that " As a means of preserving the customary, the conventional, whether in dress, habits, or ordinary usages of society, laughter stands unrivalled ", or that it confirms a conservatism which is, up to a point, an indispensable instinct for safety [60]. Now this disciplinary role of laughter, evident, admitted by all writers, and partly responsible for the belief that laughter always contains a restricted animus, depends, as directly as the humanization of laughing, upon the element of relief.

Flogging castigates with a blow and gaol castigates by confining freedom, but laughter castigates by its supercilious implication that the victim is worth neither a blow nor the trouble of confining. Thus the relief of laughter, in the very act of relaxing from aggression, hints at the foolishness or worthlessness of the person laughed at and fills him with humiliation. This wound in the spirit is often said to pierce more keenly than a wound in the body : ridicule is often a thrice-pointed lance. Thus the paradox is true : the break in aggression that initiates laughter both opens a path for sympathy and perpetuates a sharp social discipline.

The relief of laughter is the more clearly seen as a centre of growth the more completely laughter is known. Humanization and disciplinary vigour spring from it, as the varieties of laughter seem to spring from an original laughter of sheer relief. The release of opposites, like the tender sympathy of humour and the castigating contempt of disciplinary laughter, the movement of counteracting tendencies within the fundamental element of relief, is apparent in the mental sanity, geniality, and common sense conferred by laughter on the one hand and in the dangers of excess to which it exposes men on the other. The genial influence of laughter is too obvious to require emphasis, and its steadying effect on mental perspective is almost as evident. Resentment at the imputation of lack of humour is probably stirred in part by a sense of being imperfectly qualified for society by inability to join in one of its characteristic enjoyments and in part by the lack of insight that the imputation implies. If a sense of humour is the fixed associate of wisdom and implies common sense [61], an accusation of deficiency in humour is an imputation of folly. If sensitiveness to incongruities is the core of the ludicrous, comic or humorous perception is almost indispensable to sound judgment. Pomposity and dogmatism wane when men perceive the contrast between their own little pretensions and the greatness of the universe. A quiet humility descends when the fuss made by any individual is humorously contrasted with the cosmic placidity that ignores him. We cannot fit the universe, or any part of it, neatly together, as a clock-maker fits our watches ; we cannot assign man to his precise niche nor say exactly what he is nor what he should be ; and humorous perception of the incongruities in our muddled versions of things prevents us from suffering too acutely from our own failures and from presuming too much upon our own insight. Relief by laughter from the seriousness of life is a good thing, and its genial spread seems to be too great a boon to justify any warning. But laughter constantly tends to degenerate into " fun in Bagdad ". Since Plato desired the rulers of his State to be sparing of laughter, many eminent warnings have been inspired by his fears. " Persons ", wrote Hartley, " who give themselves much to mirth, wit, and humour, must greatly disqualify their understandings for the search after truth " [62]. Sydney Smith, himself a wit, perceived the probable tendency of wit and humour to corrupt understanding and heart [63]. Thomas Fuller, before them, had wisely commended

jesting where it was no "master-quality"
and only "attended on other perfections" [64].
"If the sense of the ridiculous is one side of
an impressible nature, it is very well", wrote
Oliver Wendell Holmes, adding "but if that
is all there is in a man, he had better have
been an ape at once, and so have stood at the
head of his profession" [65]. There is a tendency
to listen too eagerly for the jingle of the bells
on the jester's cap and to reward too highly
those who make us laugh. It seems ungracious to shake a warning head at eager, pleasant,
genial laughter, but the very relaxation from
which it springs is also an obvious possible
source of permanently playful idleness. Nias
hunters, when digging a pit, may not laugh
or the sides of the pit will fall in [66]. Some
taboos are founded on insight : laughter is
essentially a desistance from effort, and may
be fatally indulged. Socrates, on one occasion,
doubtless by chance and without forethought,
described the essential nature of all worthy
laughter and its essential function. When
Protarchus broke in with a laughing remark
Socrates said : "A jest may sometimes
pleasantly interrupt earnest" [67]. A pleasant
interruption : that is exactly what laughter
is ! "Sometimes" : that is exactly when
laughter should arise ! "Earnest" : that is
exactly whence the relief of laughter should
come ! Laughter is always a descent, and
when it has descended from a higher level it

will, if continued too long, sink lower and lower. For the permanent level to remain high, the descents of laughter must not be too frequent. " Laughter is open to perversion, like other good things ", wrote Meredith ; " to laugh at everything is to have no appreciation of the Comic of Comedy ", and, quoting Landor, " genuine humour and true wit require a sound and capacious mind, which is always a grave one " [68].

Relief, to summarize, is written on the physical act of laughing and on the physiological accompaniments. It is written on the occasions of laughter and, more or less plainly, on each of its varieties. A laughter of sheer relief may be the original source of all other laughters, which have spread from it like a sheaf. Humanization and social discipline are connected with laughter through its relief : relief permits sympathy to enter by ending aggression and favours a restricted animus because withholding a blow can suggest contempt. The element of relief simultaneously gives value to laughter and involves a risk of degeneracy.

Relief is not the whole of laughter, though it is its root and fundamental plan. The discovery of sudden interruption through relaxation of effort merely begins the inquiry into laughter. But it does begin it, and no discussion of laughter that ignores relief or makes it of little account can hope to prosper.

CHAPTER IV

LAUGHTER AND TICKLING

THAT familiar nursery experience, old and always new, the tickle, has left its mark on the history of theories of laughter. Joubert, remarks Mr Eastman, was wise enough to know that " any true science of humour " must include an explanation " of our pleasure in tickling " [69]. It obviously must, but the tickle must also not be too authoritative in dictating to us the nature of the ludicrous. The theories that took their cue from the tickle were, in the first place, too engrossed with the ludicrous to see quite clearly into the nature of laughter. They also assumed too readily that tickling is always pleasant and necessarily a droll occurrence. It is natural for theorists to approach laughter through amusement, or even to forget other varieties of laughter, because the sense of the ludicrous pervades laughter so freely, is prominent as a source of pleasure, and is so unique among the emotions. This engrossment with amusement, however, exacts a penalty by blinding the inquirer to the light thrown upon comic and humorous laughter by other forms. It is, perhaps, equally natural to disregard the serious side of tickling, since the nursery tickle is more familiar than any other. This second natural error again exacts a penalty by blinding inquiry to tickling that is not playful. The fact that tickling is not necessarily funny is fundamental for understanding its connection with laughter.

Tickling very seductively entices us to regard the ludicrous as a mental tickle. To say, when we laugh at a joke, that it tickled us, is almost as natural a metaphor as to call a baby " sweet ". If the " cause of laughter is but a light touch of the spirits, and not so deep an impression as in the other passions ", as Bacon said, and if laughter " is moved, and that in great vehemency, only by tickling some parts of the body " [70], it is natural to see in the violent squirm started by the lightly touching tickle an actual picture of the " happy convulsion " of laughter started by the light touch of the ludicrous upon the mind. Speaking roughly but with sufficient accuracy, the theories of laughter, mainly of comic laughter, that obviously take their cue from the tickle, study tickling as a physiognomist, who, to deduce a politician's character from his face, might, in the absence of the man, study his photograph. For such theories the tickle is a physiological imitation of laughter at the ludicrous. Now tickling seems to contain a mixture of pleasure and pain. Bacon remarks that "men even in a grieved state of mind", if they are tickled, "cannot sometimes forbear laughing": there is a pleasure in the tickle. But he adds: "and tickling is ever painful, and not well endured" [71]. Protarchus learned from Socrates that tickling is a mixture of pain and pleasure, with a greater proportion of pain [72]. Theorists have been impressed with this mingling of pleasure and pain when they have forestalled Mr Eastman's injunction to look to tickling accompanied by humorous emotion for an authentic and first picture of humour [73]. Dr Joubert, in 1579, thought that laughter "does not come of pure joy, but has some little of sadness" [74]. In tickling, he says, "the strange touch brings some pain and annoyment to the parts unaccustomed to it; but, being light it causes some kind of false pleasure, namely that it does not truly offend and that nature enjoys diversity" [75].

Thus began the development of "conflict-mixture" and "oscillation" theories. Many historical developments of thought impress the historian as inevitable, though he may think the ideas are false. The inevitableness of the comparison between the ludicrous and the tickle and the inevitable discovery of mingled pain and pleasure in tickling seem to necessitate at least one attempt to explain comic feeling as "a rapid oscillation back and forth between pleasure and pain " or as a mastery of pain by pleasure in an oscillation or struggle between them. This line of thought prevailed, mainly in Germany, during the last century [76]. It may be called, for convenience, the " tickle-theory " of laughter (more strictly, perhaps, of the ludicrous).

Though the " oscillation of feelings " may be " an interesting myth ", as Mr Eastman calls it [77], like many myths it carries a hint at the truth, as the sequel will show. The correction of the " tickle-theory " and of most explanations of the connection between laughter and tickling, is important because it seems possible to make reasonably sure of the nature of that connection. It is so difficult to analyse laughter successfully or to secure unanimity on fundamental points that anything reasonably certain about it should be clearly conceived and firmly held.

The original mistake, that encouraged thought along wrong paths, identified tickling with the tickle of nursery play. This mistake lingers still, for in 1912 a writer said " that in the phenomena of tickling we get *laughter* produced as a *purely physiological reflex*, so unconnected with mental appreciation that it has been detected appearing as early as the seventh week of life " [78]. We squirm and *laugh* when tickled, this implies, as inevitably as we close our eyes when anything moves closely to them. But laughter and tickling

44

are easily divorced. Bacon noted that " in tickling, if you tickle the sides, and give warning . . . it doth not move laughter so much " [79]. Darwin also observed that tickling is most effective when the precise point of touch is not known [80]. In affirming this retarding by " mental appreciation " these two writers repeat common knowledge. Fear, or any sufficiently strong suggestion of hostility, completes the divorce. This also is common knowledge. If you tickle a child who suspects you, and still more if he actually fears you, he will squirm but he will not laugh. Tie the victim down, bare his soles and tickle them vigorously : torture annuls amusement. The squirm of the tickled is a *struggle* : there is no struggle in laughter. Tickling may be the most crude and elementary form of play [81], but nature did not devise the tickle for the sport of children. Play often makes sportive use of activities intended for more serious purposes—as boys will wrestle and box for amusement. A closer scrutiny of tickling itself suggests that the tickle is a serious device now largely relegated to nursery play.

The playful tickle, which has so misled many, usually aims at the trunk of the body, the arm-pit, limbs, or neck. The child's bare soles also invite tickling. A careful analysis confirms the playful discovery that ticklish points are developed on the lateral chest-wall, the abdomen, the loins, the neck, and the soles of the feet [82] : the side of the waist is a favourite spot for the fingers of the tickler. The violent squirm that responds to tickling at these points in a sensitive subject is too amusing to permit, or invite, appreciation of its significance. It is so amusing and so associated with playful teasing that laughter, in the passage quoted above, was said to be as fixed in the tickle as the squirm itself. If two sets of fingers were crawled, in the manner familiar to skilled ticklers, over the waist-sides of a portly, pompous, and sensitive dignitary, the theory that wherever squirm is, laughter is, would probably be revised—perhaps, if the experiment took place on an Eastern potentate within his own territory, in gaol. The dissociableness of laughter and squirming is realized more clearly by observing the usual absence of laughter from simpler examples of tickling. "If you tickle the nostrils with a feather, or straw, it procureth sneezing", observed Bacon [83], hinting, perhaps unwittingly, that there is no indissoluble or necessary connection between tickling and laughing. Sneezing is obviously a device for ridding the nose of intrusive substances. The ticklishness of the nostrils is, equally obviously, a device to ensure the occurrence of the sneeze. The sneeze is not inherently comic, though it may provoke amusement or be jokingly provoked by a straw. The ticklish throat coughs out its intruders and the sensitive ear withdraws from the threat of intrusion, either by agitating the body, as with men, or by its own movements, as with horses. The purpose in the ticklishness of the lateral chest-wall, abdomen, loins, and neck is less obscure in the light of the tickles in nose, mouth, and ear, and a conjunction of two incidents makes it plain. A child fingers the pepper-pot, waves pepper into its nose, and sneezes violently. Touch it under the arm-pits, or finger its waist, and it wriggles vigorously. It sneezes to dislodge the pepper from its nose, and its wriggle suggests a sneeze to relieve its whole body. The violent squirm of the tickled child so obviously tries to avoid the tickling hand that, when the truth is perceived, it is difficult to understand how tickling and laughter could ever be identified or confused. Laughter neither shrinks nor advances ; tickled wriggles are violent efforts to escape. As the tickled nose sneezes to dislodge its intruder, so the tickled body struggles to dislodge the clutch of an enemy. Judging the tickle by the fun of play is like judging the sneeze by observing that it can be evoked by a straw. The ticklishness of the body, like the sneeze, is only incidentally funny. The sneeze is still useful while the squirming of the body under tickling is now largely a survival of past usefulness. This reduction to a source of play has probably helped to conceal the significance of the tickle. Now, if the ticklishness of the body is assumed to survive from a time when men and their animal ancestors frequently wrestled in fight as a device for securing violent struggling to escape, the connection between tickling and laughter seems clear.

The sneeze, the cough, and wriggling under tickle, the conclusion runs, are variants of one plan. They are vigorous actions instantly stirred by a tickle and aimed at intruders. Sneezing protects the nose, coughing protects the throat, and the tickled body struggles against an enemy's embrace. When the tickle, originally a protection against real menace, is playfully given, the situation is transformed from the seriousness of battle to the *relief* of play. The tickled child is sharply incited to resist and struggle as if he were severely threatened. Since he knows, when the tickle is playful, that he is not threatened, the situation is quite appropriate to laughter. The tickle, as the violent squirming shows, calls fiercely on the body for action and the friendliness of the attack calls action off. It is essentially a situation of *relief* and the mingling of laughter with squirming is intelligible. There is a mixture of pain and pleasure in the playful tickling of friends— here the mistaken analysts are right. They are misguided when they fail to perceive that real hostility dissipates pleasure and laughter with it.

Hartley understood that tickling is a

48

momentary pain or apprehension of it, followed by removal of the fear [84]. Sully notes that the spasm of the tickle is reflexly or inevitably provoked by the peculiar sensation of tickling, that there is an element of the unknown, and that the mirthfulness of tickling, which is affected by mood, is a transition from a momentary apprehension to a sense of harmlessness [85].

The distribution of sensitiveness over the body indicates that the tickle is primarily a device to ensure a prompt, vigorous reply to assault. Darwin noted that the most easily tickled parts are usually those least frequently touched [86]. They are least frequently touched in peace, but they are, significantly, the points of attack in war. Dr Crile pertinently observes that animals fight effectively in the dark [87] : the peculiar tickling sensations quickly warn the combatants of their opponent's grip and automatically incite appropriately vigorous struggles.

The role of the tickle is confirmed by some further observations by Dr Crile, who has clearly indicated the real significance of tickling. Since a buzzing, insect-like contact seems to tickle the ear most adequately, nature has here provided tickling specially as a protection against insects. If each ticklish spot is specialized like those on the ear, it will be most sensitive to the most probable or most dangerous attack against which it acts protectively. If there is such a distinct connection between the positions of ticklish spots and their most adequate inciters it justifies the role assigned to the tickle. Now the ribs, loins, abdomen, and neck are most effectively tickled by a *tooth-shaped* body [88]. Thus the teeth of the carnivore have deceived students of laughter who have studied it through the tickle by stimulating a curious, vigorous, and doubtless highly effective, sensitiveness to their bite on the body. This sensitiveness was so stamped in that it still persists, long after its original usefulness has waned. The violent squirm of the tickled child is an indurated relic of its remote past that now provides amusement by responding to playful hostility and by deceiving philosophizers on laughter.

The connection between the tooth of the carnivore and the squirm of the tickle is a warning to be careful to consult the past. A traveller picks up an irregular piece of metal which his experienced eye judges to be a fallen meteorite. He cuts it open and discovers a small diamond. Hatton Garden would not rave over the gem, but, pecuniarily worthless though it may be, it is a diamond. To explain its presence, the fiery passage of the meteorite through the earth's atmosphere must be consulted, when the diamond crystallized from highly heated and compressed carbon. Consultation of the past is more necessary in the realm of life than in the realm of mere matter and must not be omitted in discussing laughter. This consultation has often been neglected by students of laughter, who have not, for example, always realized how laughing has been progressively humanized as it moves towards sympathy.

To the ungracious laughters from battle-triumph to self-congratulation, the laughters of greeting or play, purely comic or humorous laughter, and to sheer laughter of relief, laughter of tickling must be provisionally added. These various laughters mingle freely, and the sense of the ludicrous, which constantly invades and tends to dominate all the others, pervades the playful tickle. Perhaps spectatorial amusement is more pronounced than the amusement of the victim. The wild struggles of the tickled child are comic because they exceed his needs : he responds to a friend as if he were an enemy. This sympathetic transference of the relief situation from participator to spectator has, as will appear in the sequel, an importance in the genesis of the varieties of laughter.

The spectatorial amusement at tickled children is usually sympathetic. Though tickling may at times be a practical joke and tinged with its malice, adults usually laugh sympathetically at the children whom they tickle without cruelty. The ready entrance of sympathy into so crude and elementary a form of humour as tickling marks the openness of laughter to it.

CHAPTER V

LAUGHTER AND PLEASURE

LAUGHTER, wrote Steele, is " a vent of any sudden joy " [89]. This adds to the rapidly multiplying varieties of laughter, or suggests its addition, the laughter of pleasure. The *New English Dictionary*, in defining the act of laughing, includes three laughters : one " produced by tickling ", one expressing a " sense of something ludicrous ", and one manifesting " mirth ". Social hilarity has been under suspicion as the mother of laughter : in the broad humour, indulgence and public gaiety of primitive communities, when the hunters had provided a feast or there was high festival after a well reaped harvest, Professor Carveth Read suggests, laughter was originally begotten [90]. The relief written on the mechanics of laughter, on its occasions and on all its associated emotions, is written on the individual hilarious mood and, almost in letters of fire, on public gaiety. That " lively din ", that " dancing in the chequered shade ", more barbarously, that

wild bacchanalian rout, looses our spirit and
we call, with Milton, on the nymph to haste

> "And bring with thee
> Jest, and youthful jollity" [91].

Temporary relief from danger or emotional
stress sensitizes the tendency to laugh, as
the German soldiers, mentioned by Herbert
Spencer, after great excitement laughed loudly
at the smallest joke [92]. When relief is complete, when the task is over or the day's
work done, when the harvest is reaped or the
hunt accomplished or the battle won, when
nothing can break the respite, then the mirthful mood descends and laughter ripples as
constantly as waves roll on a moving sea.
There may be a laughter of sheer gaiety, as
there seems to be a laughter of sheer relief,
though each gay laugh has its own special
prompting—be it the meeting of cronies, a
trifling mishap, or an incident of play. Perhaps the laughter of the mirthful mood
should be described as hilarity, as laughter at
the obviously ludicrous should be described
as amusement. Possibly, however, the mirthful mood is simply a diffused mental relief
that is a source of many laughters without
being one of them. If Steele's " sudden joy "
is momentary mirth, and mirth, as it were,
expanded and prolonged " sudden joy ",
mirthful or joyous laughing may be demanded
as an addition to the varieties of laughter.

53

But, before surrendering to this demand, since the varieties of laughter seem to be springing up like the warriors from the dragon's teeth, discretion counsels careful examination of the relation between laughter and pleasure.

An infant smiles, thought Erasmus Darwin, as a dog wags its tail—to express pleasure [93]. If the smile is an ungrown laugh and the laugh a grown-up smile, laughing presumably continues the duty of smiling by serving as the language of pleasure, and Charles Darwin regarded the expression of joy or happiness as the primary function of laughter [94]. If smiling is the natural language of pleasure in man, as Erasmus Darwin thought, and if there is no abrupt line between violent laughter and faint smiling, as Charles Darwin affirmed, laughter will probably be primarily and distinctively an expression of pleasure, and joy or happiness will be the characteristic emotion of laughing. Charles Darwin argued that the laugh is a full-grown smile because growing infants pass continuously from smiling to incipient laughter. Also, by a reversal of the original development of laughter out of the smile, gentle smiling may persist as a trace of the laughing habit [95]. Laughter begins, Freud also thinks, in the smile of the satiated nursling [96]. " Laughter ", writes Mr Eastman, " is but an addition of breath and voice and gesture to this already complicated act " of smiling [97]. This united verdict, which

54

is the spontaneous estimate of commonsense, seems to be just. If the smile steals over the infant on satiety, as Freud avers, it is a token of relaxation. Erasmus Darwin, more explicitly, says that the sphincter muscle of the mouth, after being fatigued by sucking, relaxes, and that that relaxation is visibly embodied in a smile[98]. Since the smile and the laugh are physically both expressions of relief, since the one grows gradually into the other and since they seem to be freely interchangeable, a smile on the face of one person greeting the same joke as the laugh shaking the body of another, they seem to be essentially related as more and less. A laugh is a big smile and a smile is a small laugh.

Professor McDougall fears this conclusion just because " the smile is unquestionably the normal expression of pleasure ", and accuses " both philosophers and common opinion " of " the error of confounding the laugh with the smile ". If " amusement " is the specific emotional excitement of laughter and smiling normally expresses pleasure he must obviously separate the origin and functions of smiling and laughter. The universal estimate that smiles are little laughs and laughs are big smiles is misled, in his opinion, because we often are pleased when we laugh : laughter, because it is often happy, is confused with smiling which is always happy. Laughter and smiling, he urges, must be distinct in

55

origin because they appear in the infant at different dates [99]. But so is there a difference of date between the appearance of the youth and the mature man out of the child—nevertheless they have the same origin. There is always a difference of date in development : Darwin's development of the laugh from the smile will seem to most, as McDougall admits by implication, as obvious as the stepping of the chick from the egg.

We can agree with McDougall that the " procedure very commonly adopted " of assuming " that laughter is essentially the expression of pleasure, that we laugh because we are pleased ", is a questionable assumption, without admitting his distinction between laughter and smiling, or rejecting the " pleasure-theory " of laughter because it has " given rise to two famous theories, namely— the theory of pure malevolence " and " the theory of self-congratulation "[100]. Joy, according to Descartes, can cause laughter only when it is moderate or has some wonder or hate in it[101]. He assumes, interprets McDougall, laughter to be essentially an expression of pleasure, and then attempts to explain why we are pleased with ludicrous objects. He concludes, continues the interpretation, " that it is the nature of man to rejoice at the misfortunes and defects of his fellows ", just as Hobbes concluded that we rejoice at our own immunity from these " misfortunes and

defects ". Thus " the theory of malevolence " and " the theory of self-congratulation " are the " two most famous varieties
of what may be called the pleasure theories
of laughter ". " If either of them be true ",
he adds, " laughter is essentially hateful ".[102]

If either theory is the whole truth, or most
of it, " laughter *is* essentially hateful". But
some laughters unquestionably contain malignant pleasure. The contemporaries of Pope
reviled his " misfortunes with a strange
acrimony, and made his poor deformed person
the butt for many a bolt of heavy wit "[103].
Thackeray would perceive in this coarse ridicule
both pleasure and malignance. Some laughter
is also undeniably self-congratulatory. Malig-
nancy and self-congratulatory theories mistake
a part for the whole by assuming that pleasure
at misfortune always pervades laughter because it is sometimes, and perhaps, especially
in ancient laughter, often, present. Some
laughter *is* hateful and McDougall virtually
assumes that laughter can never be hateful
without being always so.

Professor McDougall errs like the two
theories he condemns by mistaking a part for
a whole. Much, perhaps most, laughter is
amused, but not all. Though many emotions
mingle variously in laughter, and amusement
constantly pervades it, a sense of the ludicrous is not essential to the laughter of greeting and is often absent from it. Amusement

has no monopoly of laughter, any more than triumph or derision or hate or self-congratulation has a monopoly of it.

Laughter is usually pleasurable simply because the sense of relief is pleasurable. Other pleasures may contribute to the whole, amusement for example may add its own quota, but laughter is fast bound to the pleasurable because relief is naturally incompatible with the unpleasant. If this bond is ever broken it is only temporarily in abnormal or pathological laughing. But, though pleasure of relief may monopolize laughter in the sense that no laugh can normally occur without it, laughter is no monopolizer of pleasure. Mr Eastman was forgetful when he commended Darwin because he " rediscovered the obvious truth that men laugh when they are happy " [104] : they often do, but not always. " The smile is unquestionably the normal expression " of many pleasures, but not " of pleasure " [105]. When an audience is thrilled by an oratorio it does not laugh ; we do not laugh at beauty or great poetry, nor smile at the revelation of a great scientific truth. There is neither laughter nor smiling in the tense excitement of action, though exertion, like the concentration of mind on an attractive problem, may be highly pleasurable. Tense pleasure and laughter do not keep company.

A singles match is in progress on a tennis-court and a straight row of spectators watches from a raised bank at the side. As the ball flies from the left the line of heads turns with it towards the right ; as it flies from the right all heads turn with it to the left. Those heads, moving in a comical unison which is as perfectly in step as the marching of foot-guards, describe to the observer the flight of the ball on the court. If they turn in a considerable part of a semi-circle the ball has been struck over the net from one base-line to the other. If, while revolving from left to right, they halt and turn sharply back, the right-hand player has volleyed at the net. The faces reflect feeling as the moving heads are a diagram of the ball's movements. Smiles and laughter appear on the faces when a break in their rhythmic movement announces the end of a rally. The same succession of seriousness and laughing, as active play is followed by a break when a point is scored, is also apparent in the players. Neither players nor spectators laugh during the tenseness of play ; when effort moment-arily relaxes they usually all smile. The players enjoy the active periods and the spectators enjoy them too. It is clear to the philosophical observer that there are pleasures of tension and pleasures of relief. It is equally clear that laughter is as inappro-priate to the one as it is appropriate to the other.

Laughter is restricted in its expression of

joy to pleasures that contain relief. The joy that announces creation [106] does not laugh, though the creator may subsequently laugh on accomplishment. The inquirer into laughter meets relief more inevitably than Alice, when she had slipped Through the Looking-Glass, met the front-door. She could avoid it by following the apparently absurd advice of the rose " to walk the other way ". She set off towards the Red Queen and, to her surprise, instantly lost sight of her and found herself walking in again through the front-door. Then she tried the plan of walking in the opposite direction. Though " it succeeded beautifully ", the plan of searching laughter for something more fundamental or distinctive than relief fails entirely. The advice of the rose is useless here. Whatever path is trodden, whether laughter is approached through triumph or scorn or self-congratulation, whether it is studied in the laughter of greeting or the laugh of play, whether search is made in the laughter of tickling or amusement or of pleasure, however thought turns and whatever direction it follows, the quest always ends on relief. The directions pursued by our analysis have so far always ended thus and all other directions will be found to end in the same way.

A hint from Coleridge detains thought for a moment on the possibility of co-ordinating the relief essential to laughter with the belief that pleasure is the specific emotional accompaniment of laughing. "Laughter is a convulsion of the nerves ; and it seems as if nature cuts short the rapid thrill of pleasure on the nerves by a sudden convulsion of them, to prevent the sensation becoming painful"[107]. If laughter steps the intensity of pleasure down to avoid the pain of excessive strain it may be a regulatory mechanism in the general expression of joy. But violent laughter, in the very strength of its convulsions, has a high emotional excitement. When we laugh at the sudden removal of an unfounded fear, our pleasure springs out of a relief from pain, not from the reduction of an intolerable pleasure. The hint arrests, as Coleridge's hints often do arrest, but is unable to detain opinion permanently on an estimate of laughter as primarily and originally an expression of pleasure.

No single emotion or feeling seems to be the specific associate of laughter : amusement is not because, though laughter always tends to be pervaded by it, all laughing is not amused ; pleasure is not because much joy does not laugh. Unless it is desperately assumed that laughter originated as an expression of relaxation-pleasure, the situation of relief in which laughter arises must be regarded as a centre round which many feelings collect. This collection of feelings round laughter, or round the relief it expresses, and their complex mingling, explain the rich variety in laughing. If there is a specific original emotional accompaniment of relaxation-pleasure to laughter, that original laughter might well correspond to laughing from sheer relief.

A sense of rich variety in the emotional or feeling aspect of laughter has always pervaded literature. " Compare the comedies of Congreve with the Falstaff in Henry IV, or with Sterne's Corporal Trim, Uncle Toby, and Mr Shandy ", remarks Coleridge[108]. " In different persons ", thought Hartley, " the occasions of laughter must be as different as their opinions and dispositions "[109]. The varieties of laughter include in their diversity, writers constantly insist, national varieties. Coleridge distinguished the thoughtfulness of English humour from the ethereal humour of Spain[110]. The Rev. the Right Hon. Edward Lyttelton distinguishes reticent Scotch humour from the " volatile and refined, but cold " humour of the Irish[111]. A distrust of the accuracy in the analyses of national forms of humour need not deny a real sense of their differences : an observer can usually be trusted to discriminate people by a sense of their differences, though he may faultily describe their points of unlikeness. However laughters are classified, there are many to classify and many ways of classifying. Without surrendering to a classificatory passion and attempting to distinguish laughters with a fond attention to their order of genesis or other order of connection, it seems clearly and indubitably evident that a fundamental situation of relief, expressing itself physically in the act of laughing, has been a centre of collection, and also of genesis, for many mingling feelings and emotions.

It has been a centre of genesis because amusement, the sense of the ludicrous, whenever it arises, seems to be indissolubly connected with the laughable situation. This characteristic, familiar, and indefinable emotion, or feeling, is unique enough to be a formidable claimant for the specific emotional associateship, if there be such, in the combination of bodily reaction and emotion known as laughter. Amusement is peculiarly enough and intimately enough the close associate of physical laughing or smiling to prompt McDougall's theory that laughter is an instinct and amusement its specific emotional accompaniment, and to carry justification of the theory far. But the real truth seems to be that the situation provided by laughter, with its fundamental relief and often complex mingling of feelings, has provided a centre of growth for the sense of the ludicrous. Amusement is not merely relief, and analysis of the sense of the ludicrous has been notoriously inadequate, but it has sprung as a new creation, as all things that grow spring as new creations, from the fundamental situation presented by laughter.

A sheer sense of relief may be the germinal feeling of laughter. But it is wise, in studying so elusive a sprite as the spirit of laughter, to be contented with the limited degree of assurance that is possible. Amid much that is uncertain and much that is elusive the collection round the fundamental relief of laughter of many mingled feelings and the genesis of some emotions from that primary situation seem to be assured. Anger has one emotion and many actions ; laughter has one action and many emotions.

" Emotion " is here used, as before mentioned, almost interchangeably with " feeling ", to denote the affective aspect of the conscious accompaniment of laughter, without endeavouring to conform to precise definitions. McDougall has no qualms about identifying " amusement " with " emotion ", and popular impression will prefer this opinion to Bergson's dictum that emotion is a foe to laughter. Some emotions are foes, inveterate and conquering foes, to laughter : fierce anger does not laugh. But Bergson apparently does not merely mean that some emotions are inappropriate to laughter and dissipate or prevent the emotions peculiar to laughing, for he insists that laughter is usually accompanied by no feeling. " To produce the whole of its effect, then ", he also adds, "the comic demands something like a momentary anæsthesia of the heart. Its appeal is to intelligence, pure and simple " [112]. So far as this intimates a glimpse of one truth it is welcome. The dispassionate freedom of the purely comic from either animus or sympathy seems to distinguish it from the sense of the ludicrous touched with sympathy that prompted Dr Duncan to say : " I have a great regard for the Humourists, for they are generally men of a tender heart " [113]. If Bergson means that comic laughter feels *nothing*, it seems sufficient criticism to refer to McDougall's identification of the sense of amusement with emotion and to note one's next laughter at a joke. Common experience will side, if a side must be taken, rather with Herbert Spencer than with Bergson : " Strong feeling, mental or physical " is " the general cause of laughter " [114].

CHAPTER VI

LAUGHTER AND SOCIETY

WHEN a caterpillar of the *Porthesia Chrysorrhoea* butterfly is placed in a horizontal glass tube which has one end in the dark and the other in sunlight, it crawls to the lighted end. Two caterpillars placed in the dark end creep together to the light, or remain at the lighted end if they are placed there, just as either of them would do if it were in the tube alone. Three or four or five or any number of caterpillars behave precisely as one or two behave. Thus a crowd of these caterpillars is drawn by light because each individual is so drawn, and the animals are not influenced by companionship [115].

The frigate *La Belle-Poule* was searching for her consort, the corvette *Le Barceau*, after a storm had separated the two vessels. Suddenly the look-out on the frigate signalled to her crew. *All* the officers and men, thus summoned to the deck, *saw* a raft swarming with men and towed by boats flying flags of distress. A boat was lowered, manned, and rowed rapidly towards the ship-wrecked

66

sailors. As the rescuing boat approached, the rescuers saw many men clambering on the raft, *saw* them stretching out their hands and *heard* their cries of distress. But when the boat drew nearer there were no men, no boats, and no raft : there was only a drifting mass of tree-branches, covered with leaves. The shout of the look-out, comments Le Bon in telling the story, stirred a common illusion, a " collective hallucination ", in each mind. A common fear for their comrades' safety and a common hope for their discovery predisposed each member of the frigate's crew to confound drifting trees with the objects of their search. Through minds thus prepared the mistaken cry of the look-out spread as a swift, dominating suggestion [116].

When a number of human beings act similarly or think alike it is often difficult to distinguish between forces which, like light upon the caterpillars, produce common action or thought by acting separately upon each individual, and forces which, like the suggestive shout from the mast on the *La Belle-Poule*, impose community through companionship. Laughter is influenced by social contact and intercourse, but the extent and nature of this influence are difficult to assign exactly, though the extent is obviously very great. One very distinct operation upon its members by society, however, can be clearly detected in laughter.

A genius is an ordinary man greatly magnified : as Sydney Smith wrote, " The meaning of an extraordinary man is, that he is eight men, not one man "[117]. An ordinary man is a solitary man magnified by the companionship of society. This social magnification of the knowledge and powers of individuals is one of the most obvious, as it is one of the most important, effects of companionship upon human beings. Every member of a human society has more eyes than Argus : through how many eyes does he look when he reads one news-sheet ! He has more hands than Briareus : how many hands has he used when he has read a single book ! The ordinary man is the genius of the animal world, as the extraordinary man is the genius of the human, because society multiplies his knowledge and magnifies his powers.

Social contact and intercourse multiply extensively by spreading ideas, emotions, and actions among the members of groups or intensively by fixing these ideas, emotions, and actions more firmly in each individual and adding to their vigour. Social magnification distributes abroad and increases each single distribution. The shout of the look-out spread an illusion through the whole ship's company and, by spreading it, fixed it more firmly in each mind. Since this wave of suggestion, in effect, converted many observers into one highly prejudiced and completely deluded observer, Le Bon can plausibly argue that events reported by a number of persons are the most doubtful. But social magnification works up as well as down. It worked up in the boys' discussion club described by De Quincey : " What one boy had not, another had ; and thus by continual intercourse, the fragmentary contribution of one being integrated by the fragmentary contributions of others, gradually the attainments of each separate individual became, in some degree, the collective attainments of the whole senior common room "[118]. This spreading and intensifying through social contact and intercourse, which works so obviously in human societies both for weal and for woe, has operated in laughter. Monkeys smile and laugh when they are tickled or receive a tit-bit or see a friend or make friends with their keeper[119]. These simple occasions of laughter and their elementary emotions have been multiplied in man, through social influence, into a richer variety of occasions and emotions. As a laugher, as in other capacities, man is the genius of the animal world and his genius is a social product.

" The first occasion ", remarks Hartley, of children's laughter, " seems to be a surprise, which brings on a momentary fear first, and then a momentary joy in consequence of the removal of that fear. . . . This is the original of laughter in children which is multiplied by imitation. . . . For whatever can be shown to take place at all in human nature, must take place in a much higher degree than according to the original causes, from our great disposition to imitate one another " [120]. Laughter has become so important in human life because it is infectious. The encouragement of one laugh by another has spread and fixed the laughing habit, and as occasions appropriate to its fundamental nature of relief arise they find a laughing response ready prepared. As these laughing responses multiply in each person and spread through society, the tendency to laugh becomes more easily provoked and richer in variety of feeling. The first laugh of the child, usually when it is about three months old, becoming a habit as it responds to companionship and constantly attended by new emotions as the growing mind becomes capable of the various experiences that can excite laughter, hints at the development of laughter in the human race. The limited laughter of monkeys and the wider laughter of men give the same hint.

Most human actions are infectious, but some are more infectious than others. Laughter seems to be naturally well qualified for social infectiousness because its inherent relief qualifies it to express so many different

shades of feeling. Very many of these feelings, also, naturally unite men in a common
emotion : victorious triumph, public rejoic-
ings, and greetings among friends are pre-
eminently collective experiences. Relief is
too congenial and its various associated
feelings are too grateful to human hearts
and minds for laughter, which expresses so
many of them, to prefer to lurk singly.
Community is so natural to laughter that
laughing is only " without offence ", as Hobbes
remarks, when " all the company may laugh
together : for laughing to one's self putteth
all the rest into jealousy and examination
of themselves " [121]. The self-contained laugh
perhaps suggests a secret scorn, though it
may also suggest a pleasure unshared, but
even laughter of contempt can be social and
infectious, for men are often ready to share a
delight in humiliation.

Laughter is so social that it is often assumed
to have originated socially. The actual
" original of laughter " is difficult, probably
impossible, of discovery, but laughing did not
necessarily arise in social situations because
it so persistently haunts them. Hobbes, as
his critics often forget, suggested two sources
for laughter. When men laugh " they
suddenly applaud themselves " for one of
two reasons : either they compare themselves with " some deformed thing in another "
or their " grimaces " are caused " by some

sudden *act of their own* that pleaseth them " [122].
If laughter can be private, and we do laugh
privately at private thoughts, private situations may be its original source. Many writers
urge that private laughter, which has no
apparent reference to other persons, may
really contain a social situation in disguise.
Undoubtedly we are to such an extent
creatures of society that we insist, even when
we are alone, that we are really one among
many. By thinking, said Socrates to
Theætetus, " I mean the conversation which
the soul holds with herself in considering of
anything. I speak of what I hardly know ;
but the soul when thinking appears to be
just talking—asking questions of herself and
answering them, affirming and denying
them " [123]. When Socrates compared thinking,
which is private, to talking, which exchanges
ideas among many, he involuntarily thought
of himself as a group.

If there is always some subtle personification in laughter, so that a man laughing alone
and apparently at some queer thing laughs
because the thing is, though it may be unwittingly, a living or human being to his laugh,
the lone laugher always involuntarily thinks
of himself as one of a group. It is often said
that nothing can be ludicrous, or provoke
amused laughter, unless it sufficiently suggests
a social situation : when we seem to laugh at
things we really laugh because they suggest

something human. Thus a turnip will look funny if it suggests a human face. Amused laughter will probably least easily of all laughters escape from the social circle. Emerson apparently thought that even comic laughter need not be socially situated : " Separate any object, as a particular bodily man, a horse, a turnip, a flour-barrel, an umbrella, from the connection of things, and contemplate it alone, standing there in absolute Nature, it becomes at once comic ; no useful, no respectable qualities can rescue it from the ludicrous " [124]. If isolation is *per se* ludicrous, amusement probably need not imply, even unwittingly, a social situation. Angry dispute might rage over Helen Keller's sense of the ludicrous between the two opposing views. Since she was blind and dumb from birth, she appreciated the comic through touch and feelings of her own movements. The bulge of a water-melon felt ludicrous to her and she was amused at " the puffed-up rotundities of squashes " [125]. Without denying that a water-melon may amusingly suggest human pride, a physical bulge hinting at a psychical bulge, and without affirming it, there remains a presumption that comic perception need not presuppose a social situation, real or imaginary. But for laughter that arose, and arises, apart from companionship, " a sudden act of their own that pleaseth them " in the laughers, a laughter corresponding to the influence of light upon the caterpillars and free from the suggestion pervading the frigate's crew, it is wiser to search lower than amusement in some more primitive forms of laughter.

When the engine of a gramophone has been wound, a record placed on its disc and the needle placed in position, releasing the catch automatically starts the machinery and a tune is played. As the gramophone is *set* to play when the catch is released, so the body, or part of it, is *set* to wink its eyes when anything, a menacing finger for example, comes near them. In such reflex actions an external stimulus, corresponding to the released catch in the gramophone or the approaching finger in the wink, sharply prompts an action prepared in the body corresponding to the arrangement of the gramophone for producing music or the nervous mechanism to ensure winking. The term " reflex " is applied only to the responses of *living* things to stimuli. In human beings the stimulus appeals to the brain or spinal cord by an impulse transmitted through sensory nerves and the central nervous system responds by enforcing the appropriate movements through motor nerves. Sometimes the term " reflex " simply means this connection between stimulus and reaction through the nervous system ; sometimes it implies that the reaction is inevitable and uniform ; and sometimes it implies that the reaction is unconscious and involuntary[126]. Now laughter sometimes seems to happen like the tune on the gramophone when the catch is released or like winking when something moves towards the eyes.

The acridness of the *herba sardonia*, or Sardinian herb, is said to convulse the faces of those who eat it. " Sardonic ", because of this, is applied to pathological laughter in which " the nostrils are drawn upward, and the cheeks backward toward the ears ; so that the whole countenance assumes the air of a cynic spasm or sardonic grin ", or to the " involuntary, convulsive drawing down of the angles of the mouth in tetanus ". Sardonic laughter ordinarily means bitter or mocking laughter, or, as Dr Johnson put it : " what the Latins call Sardinian Laughter, a distortion of the face without gladness of heart "[127]. If the Sardinian herb automatically provokes laughter, as a finger approaching the eye automatically provokes winking, that laughter is reflex. But it hardly arises from " purely physical causes ", as Höffding seems to think[128]. The acrid taste implies an element of mental appreciation which is present in many of our reflex actions. A very large human body will jump from the point of a very small pin because there is pain in the stimulus. There is feeling in the tickling of the nostrils that ensures a sneeze, and when the eyes close before an approaching finger there is a consciousness of its approach.   None of these reflexes, sardonic laughter, shrinking from a sharp point, sneezing, or winking, are as perfectly automatic, as purely physical and devoid of consciousness, as the musical response of a gramophone to the release of the catch.

Höffding [129] mentions some other examples of reflex laughter automatically stimulated by physical causes.   A hypnotized lady burst into uncontrollable laughter whenever the bridge of her nose was pressed.   Gladiators who were wounded in the diaphragm died laughing.   Ludovicus Vives laughed irrepressibly when he first tasted food after a long fast. But none of these can be confidently affirmed to have been entirely due to physical causes, because some mental appreciation may have been present—and probably was.

Nor can an " original of laughter " purely physically provoked, like the forward leap of a motor-car without any sense of the situation when the driver moves the lever, be found in the laughter of the tickle.   Sully compromises by calling the laughter excited by tickling " quasi-reflex " [130].   If a child is tickled on the soles of its feet it will laugh only if it is contented [131] and it is clear, as already observed in Chapter IV, that in the " phenomena of tickling " laughter is *not* " produced as a purely physiological reflex " entirely " unconnected with mental appreciation ".

The laughter of the woman who was caught in machinery and threw herself on the table to laugh when she was released from the danger of mutilation or death was probably one of the most original and primary forms of laughing. Such laughter of sheer relief naturally invites this conclusion. It is most probable that a sudden, relieving interruption of *actual physical action*, involving distinct or even violent effort, was the primary occasion of laughter. The more mental occasions, when laughter more obviously " hath its source from the intellect " and there " precedeth a conceit of somewhat ridiculous " [132], most probably developed out of the more purely physical. Hobbes' hint in the " sudden act of their own " and Höffding's search for purely reflex laughters indicate the most probable originating situation for laughter. It is doubtful whether " laughter may arise from purely physical causes, and so need not be an expression of an emotion at all " [133], but it probably arose originally, and still continues to arise, in a sudden call-off from physical effort—in a relief through suddenly relaxed, because unrequired, bodily strain.

When laughter is a break in physical exertion it need not be socially situated : the woman laughed because the machine could not mangle her. Hypercriticism cannot plausibly argue that she subtly personified the machinery into a malignant demon in order to laugh. If violent cold, suddenly applied, can excite laughter [134], such laughing appears to be independent of a social *milieu*. But, without depending upon this consequence of stimulation by cold and without trusting too much to Sully's statement that " we are never affected by comicality of a thing without experiencing a tickle in the throat " [135], which suggests a relic of its original reflex nature in all laughter, it seems reasonably certain that men have laughed, and still laugh, with an emotion of sheer, unsocially determined relief. Sudden escapes from physical dangers and sudden successes in physical efforts, as when a final shove launches a boat, can provide laughters of relief and provide them without any reference to society.

The break in physical effort which provides laughter with a situation of relief can occur in fight. Triumphant laughter reveals very clearly the multiplying, intensifying and diversifying influence of society upon laughter. The sheer relief of intermitted physical action and sudden salvation from danger as the warrior vanquishes his foe has an extra emotional gusto and character because an *enemy* has been defeated. Our emotional life is most sensitive and most developed in relation to social situations. It is probably significant that sound is the most exciting sense : music is the most intensely emotional æsthetic experience that man can construct out of sense-impressions. If this fact is conjoined with the importance of the human voice in keeping psychic touch between human beings and the sensitiveness of men to one another's voices, the important role of society in stimulating and developing emotional life is manifest. Cries and words are the most important connecting links between human minds, and the emotional gusto of sounds is quite natural if society is the great source of emotion. Thus the original physical relief of laughter is exposed, in exulting triumph, to the emotional impulses incident to a social situation.

Since triumph can be shared, it spreads laughter through the group and the exultant laugh of each member becomes more exultant because it is shared. Thus in the collective triumphant laughter of a victorious tribe the original laughter of physical relief begets a social laughter in which it is spread, intensified, and developed.

Mirthful feasts of vintage or harvest or hunting contain the same core of relaxation from successful physical effort as collective battle-triumph.

The importance and primacy of successful physical effort and of actual physical relief in the situations appropriate to laughter continually tinge many varieties of laughing with exultation or triumph. The heightened sense of power after victory is prominent, Sully remarks, in primitive laughter [136]. Laughter may have originated, Professor Carveth Read conjectures, in the broad humour and indulgence after successful hunting or harvesting [137]. Mr Eastman, who thinks that unsympathetic or ungracious elements are pollutions of laughter and not parts of it, has to admit that " laughter has perhaps a more elementary—or at least a more strong and spasmodic—connection with states of triumphant lust and battle-cruelty than with any other satisfactions except those of the social instinct itself " [138]. We are actors primarily and thinkers secondarily, and, though thought may have the higher value, the ultimately active and physically striving element provides the original form for laughter, as for all experiences, and continues to give body to it. A child playing hide-and-seek who suddenly discovers a second child concealed in a cupboard laughs excitedly at its sudden success. This little incident explains gaily, as the laughing yell of triumph explains grimly, the significance of relief in physical activity for the genesis and nature of laughter.

Society freely absorbs the situation of relief so fundamental to laughter. The practical joker can actively torment his fellows and laugh over the success of his stratagems.

Play provides laughter with occasions ; scorn, contempt, and greeting provide it with more. Since his social *milieu* is man's most intimate and emotional touch with the universe, the situations of relief that invite or stimulate laughter are predominantly and almost exclusively social. Thus a laughter of sheer relief, circumspectly assumed to be the " original of laughter ", marking a break in physical effort, spread by social infection, transfused by and incorporated with a rich variety of feeling, developed into a sense of the ludicrous that seems by its peculiar quality almost to deny its kinship with other laughters, is enlarged by society till the normal civilized being collects round a fundamental centre of relief and expresses by a familiar " mechanical motion " that assemblage of feelings commonly called laughter.

Since one man can watch the success of another and laugh with him, laughter can free itself from the necessity of marking a break in actual physical effort. A solitary being who had no fellows might conceivably learn to laugh with recollected relief at a recollected achievement. However this may be, the spectatorial possibilities supplied by society were important for the destinies of laughter. When spectators of another's laughter laughed as if they had struggled and suddenly succeeded as he did, they were opening up possibilities. This spectatorial repetition in thought is accompanied by a subdued bodily imitation of the actions observed, for whenever we watch incidents or think of them we probably perform slight movements which, if they were completed, would repeat the contemplated actions exactly. Aristotle advised the poet to " act his story with the very gestures of his personages " [139] to obtain imaginative grip on his drama. Every spectator at a football match probably follows the fortunes of the game with subdued, incipient movements that imitate the movements of the players, and community of feeling in the crowd is connected with a community of action. Thus, though the spectatorial laughter which repeats the laughter of an observed action when the agent is suddenly relieved of necessity for further effort does not spring from relaxation of full physical exertion, it still retains a connection with a physical situation.

Spectatorial influence upon laughter is not limited by this sympathetic, contemplative mimicry. The man who is chasing his hat does not laugh, though he may laugh when he catches it ; the man who watches the chase does, laughter thus escapes from actual participation in an action, whether through palpable performance or mental repetition. This transference from a direct consequence of physical action to a more purely mental character represents a significant development for laughter. When Mr Max Beerbohm remarks that "the physical sensations of laughter are reached by a process whose starting-point is the mind" [140] he is noting laughter in a far remove from its original source in sheer relief when sudden success relieves physical effort. The contemplation of laughter in this far remove is apt to identify laughing emotion with the sense of the ludicrous, because amusement gradually dominates laughter as it grows away from its more elementary forms. Thus Bacon, who emphasizes, what Mr Beerbohm subsequently echoes, that "laughing . . . hath its source from the intellect", adds "for in laughing there ever precedeth a conceit of somewhat ridiculous" [141].

The original situation of physical relief, which has a mental side from the beginning, represents the fundamental plan on which all laughter is built. The perception of incongruity, which is the core of the ludicrous, is the mental equivalent in amused laughter of physical release in more elementary forms of laughing. Writers who are careful to survey laughter and note its various forms usually admit with Höffding that "laughter makes its appearance even before anything ridiculous can be realized in consciousness" [142], and with Sully that the feeling of the ludicrous is an outgrowth from more primitive forms [143]. If many feelings assemble round laughter or are expressed by it, the corresponding mental experiences will presumably have a fundamentally identical structure. The plan of this structure is most clear in the sudden relief of successful physical exertion or in a welcome relaxation of it. This original occasion, mainly through social influence, has been multiplied, extended, and modified until the physical habit of laughing, accompanied by different emotions, singly or mixed, has been stamped into the human race. Since growth seldom, if ever, proceeds in a single line, the varieties of laughter have most probably been socially educed in radiating lines from a centre of growth in sheer relief when a physical effort, because no longer required, is suddenly relaxed.

The " mechanical motion " of laughing continues the fundamental connection of all thought with physical action. When the final stroke is given, the successful striker must still act : there is nothing for him to do —so he laughs. The ludicrous situation is similar enough to this, though it may have little apparent connection with activity of body, to produce the same act of laughing.

CHAPTER VII

LAUGHTER AND CIVILIZATION

IF " the feeling of the ridiculous produces an immense effect upon human affairs "[144], human affairs also work very decisively upon laughter. Almost any human act or thought is, in principle, an index of character, and such indexes have been sought everywhere, including dreams and handwriting. One written sentence might reveal a whole character to an omniscient intelligence, as an omniscient anatomist might reconstruct a whole animal from a single vertebra. But the perfect construction is possible only if the relations between the whole body and a single vertebra are known completely, and the significance of handwriting for deducing character resembles the anatomical value of a vertebra for one who only knows that it signifies a backbone. Laughter is a more promising index, for the way men laugh and the things they laugh at reflect their tastes, thoughts, and sympathies. On a wider scale society offers its pulse in the nature of its laughter, and the fortunes of laughter reflect the movements of civilization. Laughter is a good consultant for the inquirer into human history if the consulting is discreet and conducted without forgetting that its revelation of the human mind is neither complete nor wholly intelligible.

Whether or no the " vigilant comic " is truly " the first-born of common sense " [145], which is doubtful, or " a sense of humour " necessarily " implies balanced common sense " [146], which is disputable, laughter is often a pertinent commentary on the fundamental judgments of a community. Since " common sense " is a chameleon phrase, it must be fixed to one meaning in this context. Physical position very obviously determines judgment and controls opinion. The sun seems to a watcher on the earth to move round him, and the reverse is obvious to a careful observer on Mars. In a wider sense Voltaire's Micromegas and man have entirely different standpoints : the one can creep among atoms to explore them, the other moves among grosser bodies and knows atoms only by inference. There is psychical position as there is physical position, for the estimates of any particular community depend upon its fundamental beliefs and ideas. Men's opinions vary with their general psychical standpoint. A limping Tatungolung man told Mr Howitt that an enemy had buried a piece of sharp glass in his foot-print [147]. His pre-conceptions ascribed his pains to magical influence ; Mr Howitt's preconceptions ascribed them to rheumatism. The general psychical standpoint of a community, or collection of spontaneous opinions and behaviours springing from this standpoint, is, in one meaning, its " common sense ". On this psychical position, the laughter of any community often throws a fitful light, both by the occasions that prompt it and by those that quell it.

The character and temperament of an age, as well as its common sense, are reflected in its laughter, and changes in habits of laughing are a moving index of the course of civilization. If the tooth of time had spared the " various kinds of jokes " enumerated by Aristotle in his lost " treatise on poetry ", there would have been a little more light on the manners of his time. " Some of them ", he remarks, " are suited to gentlemen, but not all ". Unfortunately only his advice to be " careful then to make use of none but such as are appropriate to your character " remains. We do know, however, that he considered irony " more gentlemanly than buffoonery "[148].

The comic warfare of the practical joke is luxuriant in *The Arabian Nights' Entertainments*. Its " mischievous adventure " revels in the deceived lover who was first beguiled into shaving his eyebrows and stripping off his clothes, then turned into a wandering passage, and finally plumped into the street through a trap-door. *The Thousand and One Nights* are full of such rough, unfeeling practical jokes that represent the manners of the East and, as Hazlitt remarks, "carry the principle of callous indifference in jest as far as it can go"[149].

The jests are too spiced with malice and the organized practical joking too obviously a comic copy of stark battle for the degree of the sense of the ludicrous in *The Arabian Nights* to be confidently appraised. How far, the inquirer asks, is there sheer glee over physical discomfiture and how far is there purely comic perception? If Hazlitt applied his scale, merely laughable-ludicrous-ridiculous[150], how would it record? Children's laughter is similarly problematic. We may be too prone to attribute to ancient mirth as sharpened a sense of the ludicrous as our own. The laughter at personal misfortunes, especially when jestingly inflicted, suggests a coarse echo of triumph in battle more than a nicer sense of the comic.

Laughter at serious discomfiture, or even at physical injury, has not absorbed sympathy any more than it is dissociated from its fundamental situation of physical action. The glee of the practical joke springs from successful action by the joker and is shared by the approving spectator. When satire substitutes mental discomfiture for physical, though it can vie with practical jesting in cruelty, it also can refine laughter and diminish its animus. One step passes from the practical joker who mauls his victim to the spectator who laughs at the mauling ; another step passes from the participating spectator to the satirist who drops physical violence out and mauls his victim mentally. In the " poetry of invective ", as Aristotle calls it, systematic satirical attack replaces the organized comic warfare of physical discomfiture. Aristotle has scattered through his *Poetics* hints at a humanization in Greek comedy. Homer, he says, outlined the general forms of comedy by substituting " a dramatic picture of the Ridiculous " for " dramatic invective ". When writers began to write comedies they soon preferred the humaner example of Homer to the coarser method. " Laughter without offence ", wrote Hobbes, " must be at the absurdities and infirmities abstracted from persons . . . " [151]. This abstraction from persons marks an extrusion of animus from laughter, and it seems clear that Aristotle meant personal satirical attack by " dramatic invective " and impersonal comic castigation by " a dramatic picture of the Ridiculous ". Thus, when Homer rejected the former and adopted the latter, he removed " offence " from laughter by avoiding personalities. Aristotle clearly traces this satirical softening in Crates, who, he says, was the first Athenian poet to frame general and non-personal stories and drop the " comedy of invective ". Without any rash deduction from Aristotle's further incidental remark that in comedy " the bitterest enemies walk off good friends at the end " he may be said to intimate plainly a humanization of organized comic laughter from personal attack to non-personal display of the ridiculous [152].

Aristotle seemed to sense an unkind tendency in the laughter of his day when he says of the young that " they are fond of laughter and *consequently* facetious, facetiousness being disciplined insolence " [153].

Fear may expel personal invective from laughter, as Dr Johnson's big stick deterred Foote from stage-caricature, and too many complex currents flow in human life for simple judgments to be safe. But other mitigations of satirical savagery have repeated the supersession of personal invective by Homer and Crates. The satire of the age of Dryden and Pope suggests a conversion of the physical buffoonery of *The Arabian Nights* into mental buffoonery. It has all the zest and all the malice of a fisticuff bout and it rejoices as fervently in humiliation or misfortune as the most brutal of practical jokes. Meredith's description of the Comic Spirit, though it may be an ideal not always attained and perhaps has more aloof coldness than human warmth, expresses the extrusion of acerbity from comedy. It does not drive, like satire, into " quivering sensibilities ", unpretentious poverty excites in it no contemptuous laugh, and its laughter is " of the order of the smile, finely tempered, showing sunlight of the mind, mental richness rather than noisy enormity " [154]. Personal invective, the satirical successor to the rough jest of physical discomfiture, steadily tends to disappear from laughter as civilization is steadily permeated by sympathy. It seems clear that vindictiveness has been progressively banished from the laugh with the march of civilization, though it clings to it still and often embitters it.

Civilization, according to Sydney Smith, improves the humour of the body into the humour of the mind [155]. The emancipation of the laugh from physical situations where actual physical violence or discomfiture of body was the prime source of the comic and other less refined satisfactions is an important element in the development of laughter. Those writers who have emphasized the influence of social *milieu* upon the fortunes of laughter assist us to realize that laughter has been no more fixed than man himself. Like man himself, like his language, like his thought, like even his emotional susceptibilities, for though his emotional equipment is one of his most unchanging characters, he is not the same emotionally as during his first days upon earth, laughter has grown and developed. Laughter has not, like the *lingula,* or tongue-shell, remained an unmoved spectator of the stream of change. Theorists sometimes forget that the central relief of laughter has made it sensitive to changes in the laughter.

Society multiplied the laughter that arose first from an interruption of physical effort in individuals by widely extending its occasions. Amused laughter, according to Sydney Smith, was similarly multiplied by that aspect of society usually described as civilization. " Civilization " is a word that must be used with a reliance on the reader's discrimination rather than on an ability to define it. Civilization improves humour, he says, from humour of the body into humour of the mind, and this improvement results from an increased demand for humour [156]. " Humour " denotes in Sydney Smith's writings, it seems right to say, " amused " laughter : it implies neither sympathy, though it may be sympathetic, nor a sense of the ludicrous dispassionately free from both sympathy and animus, nor an absence of acrimony. It is laughter at the ludicrous. He does say, in one place, that humour may be confined to instances of the ridiculous excited by character, but he adds " there *is* an incongruous not observable in character which produces the feeling of humour " [157], and the sense of his word "humour" is nearly always laughter of amusement or laughter at the comical.

Different writers differently describe the social conditions that favour the rise of laughter which is more humane, less tied to activity or posture of body, more refined and more sharpened into nice apprehension. Meredith requires for the "Comic poet" a cultivated society with quick perceptions, a community without giddiness, a period free from feverish emotion and a reasonable equality between the sexes[158]. Sydney Smith's recipe for humour is nakedly simple, unpretentious, and perhaps suggestive of sly jesting, for it is—idleness. "There are several meanings included under the term civilization : it means, having better cups and saucers than we had a century or two ago ; better laws, better manners ; and it means, also, having nothing to do,—and those who have nothing to do, must either be amused or expire with gaping "[159].

If "great persons that have their minds employed on great designs have not leisure enough to laugh", as Hobbes thought[160], Sydney Smith may have told the truth. Idleness is of two kinds, however : the one numbing, the other fruitful. It numbs when it is a permanent habit or condition. The idling habit may be so indurated as to be an actual disease. The members of one family, men and women, were content to sit for a whole day almost as motionless as statues, without reading or sewing or playing any game, even without talking. They did not sleep ; they rose to eat, and sat down again to idle ; if they thought, their thoughts are unknown. The most elementary " humour " could not grow in such a soil. But there is an idleness which is fruitful because it is a systematic part of an efficient life. A graphic passage in *Moby Dick* describes an attack upon a whale by the crew of a whaling-boat. The harpooner, upon whose skill and strength in striking the whale the success and safety of the crew depended, rowed the foremost oar. When the boat was near enough to the whale for him to cast his harpoon, his strength had been spent on his oar, and he had to seize his weapon, aim with what steadiness he could, and throw with any of his strength that remained. " To ensure the greatest efficiency in the dart ", comments Hermann Melville, " the harpooners of this world must start to their feet out of idleness, and not out of toil ". Now if by " idleness " be meant moments of relaxation, periods of *relief* that are not merely protracted inactivity, Sydney Smith hit on a truth.

Leisure in a society, like a holiday in an individual, may stir a jocund mood, and humour may spring from a diffusion of leisurely subdued hilarity, as laughter, according to Voltaire, always springs from a gaiety of disposition [161]. Hilarity, however, is not usually discriminating in its jokes, while leisured societies are presumed to be as polished in their laughter as they are in their manners. The spirit of carnival, which is hilarity at its height, has a feature in common with diffusion of leisure : it unshackles laughter. Since there is no permanent demand by seriousness, any slight call on attention is readily followed by relief, and a general happiness of mood adds zest to laughing. Hilarity laughs often and it laughs loudly ; leisured societies also laugh often if more discreetly, but the keenest laughter, which contains the fullest flavour of humour or the most intense sense of absurdity, probably arises when "great persons that have their minds employed on great designs" do find momentary leisure to laugh, or when an active community rests, like the ideal harpooner, for its next effort. Laughter, which is always a descent, is most welcome, as it is most worthy, when it falls from a height. Mr Max Beerbohm has expressed this truth by choosing to sit with Johnson at the Turk's Head instead of with Falstaff at the Boar's. "Falstaff is but a sublimated example of the 'funny man' ", and, though the agility of his mind is effectively contrasted by the massiveness of his body, Johnson's sallies have a "noble weight of character behind them" [162].

The humour of Shakespeare, as this comparison reminds us, arose in an age of adventure and achievement. A gentle, genial leisure, if it does produce more laughter than moments of quiet in vigorous action, produces it less vigorously. This vigour may become boisterousness, as hilarity is often boisterous, but vitality is always welcome, for it can be toned into strong nicety of apprehension more easily than the languid laughter of otiose repose can be stirred into vigour. There is always some danger that even laughter, like other old institutions, may die of dignity.

Whether " in the early ages of this world there was far more laughter than is to be heard now ", and whether it has simply given place to the more dignified smile[163], or has actually diminished, civilization seems to have increased and spread sympathetic laughter, and a sharpened sense of the ludicrous has probably accompanied this multiplication. Humorous laughter, in the sense of a sympathetic sense of the ludicrous, is one index of civilized habit. In the very earliest human age of the world, if society has developed an original laughter of sheer physical relief into a protean spirit, laughter was less frequent. Whether or no laughter will participate in the usual cycle of life, so observable in all that grows, and after waxing into lusty youth from a feeble beginning, mature, wane into old age, and die ; if it has become more sympathetic and more sensitive to the ludicrous, there is probably some fostering tendency in the civilization it accompanies. For laughter will be essentially what man makes it, though since reciprocity pervades life, man will also be, in some measure, what laughter makes him.

Any community, writes Professor Flinders Petrie, has civilization when it lives justly, securely, tolerantly, and with knowledge [164]. These four qualities are connected. Men feel secure if they know they will be treated justly ; when they have security against injustice they can be tolerant, though they do not always tolerate ; though knowledge is power and is often abused, it does steadily promote the humaner traits in mankind. The emphasis for the present discussion must fall on " security ". If Sydney Smith's recipe of " idleness " is modified into " security ", to which it is akin though not identical with it, the humanizing influence of civilization upon laughter seems to be disclosed. Though laughter is less a positive act of " joyous surrender " than a spontaneous token of freedom, it requires some sort of liberty. It arises essentially in a situation of relief. When belligerency rules, the laugh is naturally an expression of triumph as the foe is disarmed or slain, or of contempt for a menace that is impotent. Belligerent laughters of different grades, from battle-triumph to unkind jesting, will naturally prevail when a latent enmity pervades a rough-and-tumble society. As security grows, doubly provided by actual social coercion or the strong arm of the law, and by the restraint flowing from good feeling and fellowship, since provocation is less, the hostility of laughter is less too. As the situation of relief that results in laughter becomes less frequently freedom from hostility, it will naturally result in more genial laughter. Men still struggle with one another; they still wage fierce wars; and they still compete in politics, in trade, in industry, in providing entertainment, and even in talk. There are still competitive elements to tinge the situation of relief, and thence to tinge laughter with superiority and even with contempt or triumph. But civilized men have learned both to subdue their hostilities and to submerge them in fellow-feeling. The result is apparent in their laughter, for laughter distinctly seems to be more kindly, as it also seems to be more distinctly sensitive to the ludicrous, in the amusement of the new world than in the amusement of the old.

There may be, it seems almost certain that there is, a connection between civilized width of knowledge and the sharpening of the ludicrous sense. The comic sense develops in the child as its experience opens its mind to the perception of those incongruities that are the soul of the ludicrous. Many writers agree upon this. Infancy and childhood offer historical hints, though children do not meticulously repeat the story of their race. The same growth of comic perception as occurs in the child seems to be evident in the growth of the human race. In one aspect the development of knowledge and experience is a growth in discrimination, and a growth in discrimination would seem to be naturally associated with a more delicate perception of incongruities.

International turbulence must not be allowed to deceive us into believing that civilization has resulted in no humanization. Civilization has increased the security that flows from mutual goodwill, though it has not made all men into friends. This increase of mutual security through fellowship is reflected in a humanization of laughter. Civilization has also widened human minds, though there is much widening yet to do. This widening, with its associated increase in discrimination, has sharpened the sense of the ludicrous and profoundly modified laughter.

CHAPTER VIII

LAUGHTER AND THE LUDICROUS

THE situation of relief in which laughter arises and from which its emotional quality is received according to the nature of the relief is also a source of a specific and pervasive emotional colouring that constantly diffuses through laughing and tends to dominate it. Relief is a break, and the two sides of the break constitute an incongruity. The sense of the ludicrous has been connected by a large company of writers with a perception of the incongruous. The great unanimity of this verdict suggests one definite step in analysis. A single disclosure of feature under scrutiny, though only one step in analysis, is still an advance. Even when the power of the poppy was merely ascribed to a " soporific principle " fruitful analysis began. There is a difference between sedative or narcotic efficacy lodged in the whole poppy and that lodged in a part of it. When chemistry followed the clue of a " soporific principle ", it discovered morphia and its associated alkaloids ; when it learned

how to assess medicinal value by assaying
the alkaloidal content of opium, it justified
the fruitfulness of assuming a " soporific
principle ". The simple recognition of incongruity in ludicrous things or situations
may be similarly fruitful though it seems a
meagre result of much thought. The combination of relief and incongruity on which
amused laughter finally depends advances
analysis a little further. Even if the result
is still meagre, and most writers sympathize
yet with Quintilian's plaint that many trials
have failed to explain satisfactorily what
laughter is[165], it is important to hold firmly
to what can be known. The sense of the
ludicrous appears to originate in the appreciation of an incongruity that forms, as it were,
the two sides of a situation of relief. Amusement, in its sense of laughter at the ludicrous,
is a familiar, unique, and prevalent emotion ;
it may be, in itself, indefinable like all emotions, and only analysable, so far as it is analysable, again like all emotions, by describing
its occasions. These occasions appear to be
situations which are broken into incongruities by sudden relief.

Unfortunately, the original source, " original" in a literary sense and as far as any source
is perfectly primary, of analyses of the ludicrous has been largely dried up. Aristotle's
separate treatment of " humour " has been
lost, and only the hints he has scattered

through his extant writings, mainly in the *rhetoric* and *poetics*, remain. The *locus classicus* of Aristotle's theory of the ridiculous runs thus : " As for Comedy, it is (as has been observed) an imitation of men worse than the average ; worse, however, not as regards any and every sort of fault, but only as regards one particular kind, the Ridiculous, which is a species of the Ugly. The Ridiculous may be defined as a mistake or a deformity not productive of pain or harm to others ; the mask, for instance, that excites laughter, is something ugly and distorted without causing pain " [166]. This passage recognizes the double factor of incongruity and relief in the ludicrous. The ugly disturbs what would otherwise be the order, symmetry, rhythm, and harmony that Aristotle assigns to the beautiful [167] : mistakes and deformities are incongruous with their context. The comic mask calls the mind to attention : inciting curiosity to stir the mind and prepare the body for action, for the possibility of a demand on physical effort lurks in all moments of mental tension, since the mind was primarily developed to participate in bodily behaviour towards persons and things. The sharp call contains a hint of menace, or, at least, of an occasion for decision and action, as all sharp appeals to the mind, because of the fundamentally practical nature of life, contain it. Then the mask is realized as a show without substance—the tension falls, and relief follows. The absence of pain and danger permits relapse into relief, and the sharp contrast between the appearance of danger and assurance of safety stirs a sense of the ludicrous. Aristotle may have thought of the incongruities in the mask itself as well as of the incongruousness diffused through the whole situation. A large nose on a comic mask rouses the mind to contemplate a large face ; the unexpectedly diminutive face requires less than anticipation expected and an appreciation of incongruity permitted by relief again stirs a feeling of the ludicrous.

Coleridge's paraphrase of Aristotle runs : " I think Aristotle has already excellently defined the laughable, τὸ γελοῖον, as consisting of, or depending on, what is out of its proper time and place, yet without danger or pain." The impropriety, he adds, is the positive, and the dangerlessness the negative, qualification[168]. This circles round an analysis of amused laughter as a sharp sense of incongruity, the impropriety, permitted by, or suffused with, relief, the sense of dangerlessness. Incongruities too strongly spiced with menace, when a call of sensed danger drops, may hinder the flow of ludicrous feeling. The whizz of an arrow past the ear favours an emotion of relief more than a grin at the fun of the thing. Whether Aristotle considered the dissipated menace of the mask chiefly

important, or not, for the ludicrousness of the
situation, he knew that the ludicrous does not
require a situation spiced by menace. " And
the same is true of what Theodorus calls
' novel phrases ', *i.e.* phrases in which the
sequel is unexpected and not, as he expresses
it, ' according to previous expectation ', but
such as comic writers use when they alter
the forms of words. The effect of jokes
depending upon changes of letters is the same ;
they deceive the expectation. Nor are these
jokes found only in prose—they occur also
in verses where the conclusion is not such as
the audience expected, *e.g.*

> And as he walked, beneath his feet
> Were—chilblains,

whereas the audience expected the writer to
say sandals." The " deceived expectation ",
destined for fame in many later theories of
laughter, thus stepped into its role in the very
beginning. It obviously contains an incongruity. Aristotle also hints distinctly at the
element of relaxation in the sense of the
ludicrous. " Similarly, as amusement and
relaxation of every kind and humour are
pleasant . . . ": humour is implicitly included
among situations of relief. " We are placable
when we are in such a condition as is opposed
to angry feeling, *e.g.* at a time of sport or
laughter or festivity or in the enjoyment of
prosperity or success " [169] : the relief in

laughter is exposed by contrast with the tenseness of anger and suggested in the enumeration of its associates.

These hints scattered by Aristotle can be constructed into a deceived expectation dropping into relief. The sense of the ludicrous also perceives the deceit as an incongruity. In amused laughter deceived expectation is also relieved and an incongruous contrast is perceived.

All morally wrong actions can be conveniently regarded as varieties of stealing. Deceit, for instance, is robbing people of truth and calumny takes away their reputations, as literal stealing deprives them of a material possession. If this method of statement is neither pressed too far nor taken too literally, it gives a convenient mental grip on moral wrong. The many provocations of the sense of the ludicrous can be similarly regarded as different ways of deceiving expectation, for convenience of mental grip and without insisting on the literal truth of the assertion. The converse of the proposition that every ludicrous situation practises a deception on expectancy is not true, and Aristotle, no doubt, knew that news of defeat when victory is expected is not laughable.

If expectancy of mind is compared to the physical preparation of body which precedes each action, like the bracing of muscles before lifting a weight or the constantly changing poses of a tennis-player as he makes his strokes, a deceived expectation is analogous to the arrest of a prepared action. The ludicrously incongruous is a break in the smooth flow of attention, comparable to the relief that breaks the continuity of action. The break, in either instance, may be rapid, the summons to attention or effort being promptly called off, or it may be deferred. The sense of the ludicrous springing from the mental interruption of attention corresponds to the sense of relief springing from interruption of physical effort or of preparation for it. The sense of sheer relief that has been assumed to represent the physical situation is mental or conscious in the wide sense. But the sense of interrupted mental attention is lodged, so to speak, more in the heart of consciousness and the sense of the ludicrous arises and becomes keener as the situation becomes more purely mental by removal from the sphere of the physical. When Bergson assigns, as conditions for the rise of the comic, the imposition of silence on emotion and exclusive play for intelligence[170], he probably thinks of the *perception* of incongruity contained in the sense of the ludicrous. There is not merely a break in the flow of verified expectancy, as there may be a feeling of break in the continuity of action, nor merely a break, but an apprehension by intelligence that a break has occurred. The sense of the ludicrous certainly seems to have a characteristic emotional accompaniment which can be connected with the incidence of the break, corresponding to the sudden relaxation through interrupted effort which is not needed—to relief.

In the illustrative lines quoted by Aristotle the hearer's attention, directed by the words, runs smoothly with constantly verified expectancy until the word "chilblains". The check, at this point, ceases to require devotion from expectant attention and no other effort is required from it. Expectancy is both unverified and satisfied—the purely mental situation thus corresponding to a relief of physical effort. If expectancy is diverted from one preparation of attention to another of greater, or even equal, seriousness, the ludicrous sense is stifled at birth because there is break without relief.

Herbert Spencer expressed this fundamental necessity for relief in the ludicrous break in expectancy by describing the occasion of laughter as a " descending incongruity ". A sneeze in the middle of Beethoven's symphony releases the audience " from an irksome attitude of mind " [171]. A flow of serious expectancy, not necessarily "irksome", follows the demand of the music ; then it is suddenly unverified, the sneeze satisfies attention for the moment, relief blends with a perception of the incongruous sides of the break, and a laugh, expressing relief and charged with a sense of the ludicrous, spreads through the audience.

" The effect of contrast ", writes Höffding, " on which the ridiculous depends, results from the conjunction of two thoughts or impressions, each of which excites a feeling, and the second of which razes what the first erects " [172]. This might be a little homily on a text taken from a declaration by Kant that laughter appears when an expectation suddenly ends in nothing [173]. The expectation must really end in nothing or, perhaps more accurately, in something satisfying that does not spur attention. A sense of frustration or disappointment will quell joy and destroy amusement. It seems preferable to say that the deception of expectancy must end in relief.

When Prospero was praising Miranda he forestalled Ferdinand's smile by exclaiming : " she will outstrip all praise ". Prospero armed himself too anxiously against absurdity, for Ferdinand had too much lover's ecstasy to suspect exaggeration in praise of his mistress. A cooler auditor might have smiled because exaggeration, real or fancied, tends to be comical. An angler tells a listener that he has caught a very large fish. The listener is expectant. " It was so big that "—the listener is on tiptoes—" when I pulled it out the level of the water in the lake sank two feet "—expectation is disillusioned and the listener laughs. Exaggeration deceives expectancy by enticing it up higher than it should go. When the fraud is discovered, promise and performance incongruously contrast, attention relaxes, and amused laughter results. The fraud must be soft enough for amusement to be a sufficient recompense—the exaggerative deceit must end in relief.

Understatement entices expectation to dispense with a belief. Discovery of the deceit again incongruously contrasts reality and appearance. If the mind is satisfied with the position from which it has been anticipatively enticed, relief makes the deception laughable.

Aristotle's distinction between looking up to the characters of tragedy and looking down on those of comedy [174] suggests a " degradation " theory of the ludicrous. A drunken man is funny because he traverses human dignity. Degradation implies deceived expectation : we expect the drunkard to behave like a man, and discover that he behaves like a sot. If the mind can rest satisfied in the descent from serious expectation of dignified human behaviour, relief and incongruity combine into amusement. Relief is obviously necessary because, if it is destroyed by disgust or condemnation or pity, the drunkard is not ludicrous. Drunkenness, like physical deformity, is being unfrocked as an occasion of laughter. It steadily tends to provoke only the more uncouth varieties of laughing. The humanization of laughter is clearly reflected in a marked dissociation of the ludicrous from the degrading. Pope aimed at a ludicrous effort by a reminder that prisoners in Bridewell were flogged after morning prayers [175]. " To most minds ", comments Bain, " the ludicrousness of the conjunction would be overborne by another sentiment " [176]. There is no relief for a humane mind in this incongruous conjunction. Laughter is sensitized to human sympathies and preferences through its relief, and situations will provoke laughter or fail to provoke it as the mind can settle comfortably into the relief they provide or not.

Harmless discomposure of dignity is, however, still fruitful in laughter. Mr Edwin A. Ward had painted a portrait of Mr Scott, the chairman of the National Provident Institution, and the portrait was presented after a complimentary dinner. During the dinner the portrait was veiled. Before the unveiling, Sir Thomas Chambers, Recorder of the City of London, made a speech and asked Mr Scott to accept the gift of his portrait. As all eyes turned to the concealing curtains every mind expected " the picture of a dignified old gentleman of seventy-seven years ". The falling curtains disappointed this expectancy of dignity, for the old gentleman was " stand-

ing on his head, with his legs in the air " [177].
The sudden check to expectancy, simply
produced by inverting a picture, could drop
from its summons to contemplate dignity
into a condition of relief. No personal mischance disturbed the ludicrous situation by
calling for active sympathy, and relief united
with perception of incongruity in a volley of
amused laughter. Such laughter need contain no hostility, nor need the laughers
applaud their own exemption from loss of
dignity. The laughter of such a company,
indeed, when all were presumably in sympathy
with the subject of the vicarious indignity,
was probably humorous in the sense of amusement suffused with sympathy. It united
victim and friends in a common feeling of
kindliness sharpened into keen enjoyment by
a common zest in a ludicrous situation.
There is no contradiction between saying that
no restraint was imposed on laughter by sympathies for mischance and saying that a
suffusion of sympathy converted purely comic
laughter into humorous. Though the occasion
called for no pity for misfortune, it excited the
general sympathetic rapport between all
members of the company.

The picture might have been deliberately
inverted as an insult. A suspicion of this
would check laughter in the subject of the
joke, and animus would tinge the triumphant
laughter of the successful joker. A secret

enemy in the company would, in any event, mix triumph with his amusement. The relief of the secret enemy would end deceived expectation on satisfied animus. If the subject of the joke suspected insult, his checked expectancy would be simultaneously solicited to contemplate animosity, and there would be no relief in the perception of incongruity. These possibilities reveal the sensitiveness of the incongruous situation to the total condition of the mind, and, it may be added, in terms of general parlance, of the heart. Laughter, to repeat, is sensitized through its element of relief to its *milieu*, whether personal or social.

Great pretensions excite great hopes and inspire expectancy with respect. Pompous, inflated language opens like a trap-door under expectation, even as it stirs it with hope, and precipitates it into disillusion. The comic laugh then peals easily, for pompous promise and lean performance are in ludicrous contrast and the mind is eased from effortful understanding. Swollen phrases that excite expectancy by pretending to be big with meaning become instantly laughable when they collapse into a description of ordinary things. Don Armado had a habit of inviting ridicule by adding the plain meaning to define its own grandiloquent phrases. "Sir, it is the King's most sweet pleasure to congratulate the Princess at her pavilion in the posteriors of this day, which the rude multitude call the afternoon "[178]. When the mask is torn from the hypocrite, laughter has a great moment. Systematic hypocrisy has secured a perpetual tribute of respect, and when expectancy turns towards the hypocrite it is highly charged with hope ; as the mask falls the relapse from honour to disgrace throws expectancy from such a height that sharp contrast and deep relief prompt an irresistible sense of the comic.

The fundamental model on which all laughter is built is a situation broken into incongruity by relief. In sheer laughter of relief perception of incongruity plays a minimum part. When laughter is purely comic, when amusement fills it entirely up, relief plays the minimal part and perception of incongruity the maximal. The dependence of the jest's prosperity upon the ear depends, in purely comic laughter, upon how incongruities strike the mind behind the ear. The geometrical figure of a tangent touching a circle does not naturally suggest itself to most people as an apt illustration of the ludicrous. Yet Schopenhauer chose it [179] to illustrate his theory that laughter expresses a sudden perception of an incongruity between our conceptions of objects and the objects themselves [180]. On Schopenhauer's theory, since we expect to find in objects what we think they contain and find they do not, expectation is deceived in amused laughter. We expect an angle where the tangent touches the circle, and there is no angle, because the circling line is curved. Absence of relief is no hindrance to laughter here—to most people the hindrance would be absence of incongruous prompting to the comic. But Schopenhauer's perplexing illustration has one very important significance. His amusement at this geometrical figure must have been as pure an example of wholly comic laughter as it seems possible to find. Here, if anywhere, Bergson's laughter of pure intelligence would be found. The sense of amusement appears to contain feeling for the ludicrous even when it bubbles up at the sight of a straight line touching a curved one. But it could hardly be suffused or mingled with any emotion that would be appropriate to a social situation. The deceptive angle, or non-angle, invites neither condemnation for false pretences, nor triumph over the discovery of its deceit, nor union in kindly sympathy with the laugher. If Schopenhauer chose the tangent and circle as a laughable instance, he was amused at it ; if he was amused, he laughed with wholly comic laughter ; if his joy was wholly comic, there exists, though it is seldom naked, a pure sense of the ludicrous, dispassionately free from animus on the one hand and from sympathy on the other.

As Schopenhauer chuckles quietly over his diagram we may laugh quietly at him for chuckling. The situation at once attracts contemplative inquirers. Bain might reflect that possibly " laughter can be excited . . . against . . . inanimate things that " have *not* " contracted associations of dignity " by " personification ". He might also wonder whether " the occasion of the ludicrous is " *always* " the degradation of some person or interest possessing dignity, in circumstances that excite no other strong emotion " [181]. We have already concluded that laughter probably did not arise in a social situation and probably does not necessarily require to personify its inanimate objects. Is Schopenhauer unwittingly accusing his non-angle of deceitfulness, as if it were human ? Aristotle notes that the philosopher expected an angle and did not find it. Kant might be doubtful whether Schopenhauer's expectation had dwindled to *nothing*. Campbell would exclaim to theorizers who identify laughter with scoffing " there is no contempt in this geometrical joke " [182]. Bergson can hardly persuade us that the quiet chuckle is pure intelligence empty of emotion : Schopenhauer is *amused*—he does not merely perceive a non-angle where an angle should be.

Our own laughter seems to be humorous. We can hardly despise Schopenhauer for extracting a joke from a bald bit of geometry, and there seems to be a link of sympathy between him and us. One of the inquiring circle has denied that humour is simply " a lively sense of the comic tempered by kindly feeling ", and defined it as " a more subtle, delicately discriminating sense of incongruity "[183]. But Schopenhauer seems to hint distinctly at a purely comic sense, which may be sharply discriminative of incongruity, into which amusement, a sense of the ludicrous, and no other emotion, enters. When we laugh at the naïveté of a child, amused at the contrast between its immaturity and the maturity to come, sympathy seems to pervade our laughter. Our laughing binds him to us. This seems to be humorous laughter. Nice, appreciative discrimination of incongruity is cold, as all purely intellectual operation is cold. Even the sense of amusement which throbs in comic perception has not the warmth of human sympathy that we seem to discover in humorous laughter. George Eliot allows " a high degree of humour to practical jokes," and defines only higher forms of humour " as the sympathetic presentation of incongruous elements in human nature and life "[184]. " Humour " here means amusement or sense of the ludicrous : in practical joking it co-operates with animus or the spirit of successful attack : it is sympathetic in higher forms which correspond to " humour " as the word is used in this book. The word " humour " is now used very generally to denote any laughter at the ludicrous, and many writers mean by it any kind of laughter whatever.

" Humour " is thus used to-day to mean the sense of the ludicrous, amusement, and usually implies that all laughter is essentially amused. But if relief is fundamental in the laughable situation the varieties of laughter are not merely different methods of greeting the ludicrous [185]. Triumph is *part* of triumphant laughter, as contempt is part of contemptuous laughter. The pure laughters of greeting or of play seem to contain, *per se*, no comic or ludicrous sense. Delight in physical discomfiture seems to be the major element in coarse practical joking and horseplay. Hilarious laughter is often but lightly touched with comic perception. If the cruder laughters are but methods of greeting the ludicrous, they are clumsy machineries for the purpose. Laughter so laden with feelings other than amusement itself can hardly be a reaction specifically appropriated and originally arising to express the sense of the ludicrous. If relief is the primary fact in laughter the sense of the ludicrous, which depends upon intellectual apprehension of the incongruity in the break by relief, will be the later comer and will tend to pervade every form of laughing. The mechanics and physiology of the physical act of laughing affirm, and examinations of the occasions of laughter confirm, the primacy of relief in laughter.

The character of any laugh depends on the

fall of emphasis in the situation. In sheer laughter of relief the emphasis falls on the break ; in purely comic laughter it falls on the perception of the incongruity forming, as it were, the sides of the break. In triumphant laughter the satisfaction of victory predominates. There is opportunity for comic appreciation in these violent forms of laughter, since there is incongruousness in the quick change of situation, but the ludicrous sense has most opportunity in less stormy varieties of laughing. The insistence by some writers on the mental sources of laughter and Bergson's exaggerated estimate of the comic sense as devoid of emotion have sensed the quietened " mechanical motion " that is associated with ludicrous perception. Laughter tends to quieten, as it tends to refine, when it passes from the service of coarser emotion to the service of the comic. Comic perception has crept steadily into laughter as history has rolled on. Humanization of thought and feeling, by forbidding vindictive occasions and expelling vindictive elements from laughable situations, has fostered laughter at the ludicrous. The rise in security from vindictiveness, as civilized men feel safer because social repression and diffusion of mutual good will diminish aggressiveness, encourages inoffensive laughter. It is quite possible that civilized sharpening of the ludicrous sense may disturb our apprehension of much ancient mirth, and perhaps of some modern.

We may misread ludicrousness into jollity
or jocular aggression. Ruder laughters may
be more purely uproarious paeans of mimic
jesting warfare than our preoccupation with
amused laughter allows us to perceive. Now,
since laughters are various and contain the
sense of the ludicrous, when it is present, in
many different settings, it seems right to
single out humorous laughter as a variety in
which comic perception is combined with
links of sympathy among the laughers. When
one person laughs simultaneously at and with
another, and especially if there is more "with"
than "at", his laughter, and indeed the
laughter of both, seems to deserve the special
title of "humour". Comic laughter, then,
is amused laughter containing feeling of the
ludicrous. It may be pure, and when thus dispassionately free from animus or sympathy is
comic laughter *par excellence* ; it may be mixed
with triumph or contempt or other emotions,
and, according to predominance of feeling, may
be classed as triumphant, contemptuous, and
the like. When amused laughter participates
sympathetically in the ludicrous situation it
can be properly described as "humour".

Bain considered humour "something genial
and loving", and, though he affirmed "an
element of degradation" in all humour, even
the most genial, "the indignity is disguised,
and, as it were, oiled, by some kindly infusion,
such as would not consist with the unmiti-

gated glee of triumphant superiority"[186]. Bain does not shut his eyes to the constant hankering of the laugh after the closed fist. Writers who recognize clearly the development of laughter and allow for it in their exposition usually regard humour as sympathetic laughter. In the mixed feeling of humour, according to Sully, "crowing" laughter is further softened and disguised by an admixture of feelings giving worth to the object and more especially affection and sympathy[187]. Sully does not forget that the competitive spirit is too much abroad in human life for laughter to escape easily from it. "The feeling of the ridiculous", writes Höffding, "with a substratum of sympathy is what is called humour"[188].

There is clearly an inclination to define humour as a sympathetic sense of the ludicrous and, equally obviously, a reluctance to admit that laughter is ever, in the full sense, humorous. If comic laughter were ever full of sympathy and completely purged from every relic of animus, interpretation of opinion might run, it would be humour. The varieties of laughter mingle very freely, and pure humour is perhaps relatively scarce. But laughter is often humorous enough to justify the discrimination of humour as a definite species of laughter. The source of amused laughter is an incongruity that deceives expectation and drops attention into relief; humorous laughter adds sympathetic linkage to perception of the comic.

Precise definitions are lacking in the terminology of laughter and terms are used somewhat indiscriminately. The word " jest " perhaps sounds more harshly than " joke " in some ears because it suggests a traditional connection with roughness and foolery. But different writers probably sense the difference, as they may do also in other instances, differently. Some may regard the words " ridiculous " and " ludicrous " as equivalents, and perhaps add that the former is displacing the latter. The use of " ludicrous " in this book has relied on the intuition of the reader and must continue to rely on it. It does not mean either derisive or humorous laughter, as its meaning is alternatively given in *The New English Dictionary*. This will now be clear. *The New English Dictionary* favours the use of " ridiculous " to express the acme of ludicrousness and this, with a qualification, is probably the best way to use the word. There must be a qualification because the notion of the preposterous, which attaches to excessive ludicrousness, implies something logically absurd. It seems possible and right to reserve the word " ridiculous " for a combination of the sense of the ludicrous with a logical condemnation. The purely comic or purely ludicrous need arouse no comment— the experience is amusing and provokes sheer comic emotion. A ridiculous statement is ludicrous and false—ludicrous in its falseness or false in its ludicrousness, as you will.

Hazlitt distinguished the " merely laughable "
as " an accidental contradiction between our
expectations and the event ", from the
ludicrous, where the contradiction is " heightened by some deformity or inconvenience ",
and both from the ridiculous in which as
" the highest degree of the laughable ", there
is a departure from common sense and reason
and not merely from custom [189]. This agrees
fairly well with a definition of the ridiculous
as a ludicrous exposure of foolishness, and the
history and present usage of the word con-
forms well to this meaning. The ridiculous,
then, when the word is used advisedly,
should mean both ludicrous and silly.

One word usually included in the vocabulary
of laughter troubles the theorist. Traill [190]
contrasted the display of incongruity by
humour with the revelation of an unsuspected
similarity by wit. This definition of wit is
very usual, and it seriously disturbs the
serenity of the conclusion that amused laughter
is necessarily prompted by an incongruity.
If witticisms flourish on congruencies and are
ludicrous, the relief-incongruity theory of the
comic may survive as an explanation of
amused laughter, but it will obviously require
ingenious manipulation. The sequel will
avoid this ingenious manipulation by denying
that wit, *as such*, is amusing. It will also
modify Traill's definition, though, since wit

certainly flourishes on comparisons without always requiring them, this modification is not so relevant to the major issue.

A preliminary hint of the relation between wit and comic laughter will be a convenient finish to the conclusion that amused laughter always depends on a situation presenting both incongruity and relief. An aggressive witticism, like the sword-stroke that ends a fight, produces a sudden relief. So does the illuminating witticism that reveals a truth. The relief is not the wit, as the relief of victory is not the sword-stroke that secures it. Wit also incidentally results in incongruities. Amused laughter can arise from the relief and the incongruities in close connection with wit without being part of it. This hint will indicate that the frequent conjunction of wit and amused laughter need not be fatal to the relief-incongruity theory of the ludicrous, though further justification must now be given.

Traill thought that laughter often accompanies wit because dissimilarities are simultaneously exposed by the witty revelation of similarities. This opinion, which is implied in his description of humour as a display of incongruities and the sole excitant of laughter, affirms a connection between the witticisms and the joke similar to, though not identical with, the connection now to be discussed.

CHAPTER IX

LAUGHTER AND WIT

THE word " wit " has fallen upon thieves, who have stripped it and forced it to masquerade in borrowed meanings, or more properly perhaps, it has suffered in meaning and reputation through the company it has been compelled to keep. One source of its misfortunes has been a confusion between the witticism and the joke. Wit has been mistakenly regarded as part of laughter, and the word is now used, in common speech, very indiscriminately to denote anything humorous or funny. In describing pantomime-patter the word " witty " is often used as an almost equal alternative to " humorous " or " funny " or " comical " : the speaker's memory being, as it were, a lucky-bag from which he takes whichever word comes first to hand.

Unless " wit " is frankly abandoned to this widened usage and no attempt is made to reserve its original meaning for it, this identification of wit with amused laughter confuses close neighbours with family inmates. For wit, as formerly conceived and as its tradition still persists, is a double achievement of insight and expression. It illuminates a truth suddenly and vividly, as a house covered by darkness is revealed by the sweep of a searchlight. " Their only means of government ", exclaimed Grattan, " are the guinea and the gallows ". Wrote Vauvenargues : " Great thoughts come from the heart ". The insight of wit may vary from a master-truth of human life to an exposure of political imperfection. Since it may also be dedicated to trifles and truisms, and since all expression of insight is not witty, its essence lies in the suddenness and vividness of its revelation. All revelation, however, must reveal something, though that something be humble, and high wit has deep insight, its achievement, therefore, may be considered " double ". The degradation of the term " wit " to denote the sallies of nimble fancy that are more entertaining than wise, which has accompanied its reduction to a species of the amusing, is intimated in Lord Morley's use of the term " aphorism ". Sydney Smith wrote of Sir James Macintosh : " New and sudden relations of ideas flashed across his mind in reasoning, and produced the same effect as wit, and would have been called wit, if a sense of their utility and importance had not often overpowered the admiration of novelty, and entitled them to the higher name of wisdom " [191]. Lord

Morley appropriated such "wisdom" to the aphorism which compresses a mass of thought and observation into a single saying [192]. The aphorism may assist to lower the dignity of wit by relieving it of its more serious significance. Its inclination towards soberness and seriousness was ready to restrict wit to a more volatile role. In its youth, wrote Bacon, knowledge "is in aphorisms and observations" [193]. Such aphorisms must contain "the pith and heart of sciences" and be filled with "some good quantity of observation". They test "the writer, whether he be superficial or solid", they are "fit to win consent or belief", and, since they represent "a knowledge broken", they "invite men to inquire farther" [194]. Johnson extolled "the excellence of aphorisms . . . in the comprehension of some obvious and useful truth in a few words" [195]. Whether the aphorism compresses into one single saying the matured insight of research, as when Bacon regards it as a pithy expression of scientific principles, or concentrates common sense wisdom into a phrase, as Johnson thinks of it, it tends to deprive wit of its higher offices and to restrict it more or less severely to mere nimbleness of fancy.

The tendency of wit to brilliant trifling, and, it may be added, to speaking daggers, is connected with its predilection for Aristotle's maxim for poets : "but the greatest thing by far is to be a master of metaphor " [196]. Metaphor inclines to comparisons, and comparisons are very usual search-lights of wit : " Experience is a good schoolmaster, but the school-fees are somewhat heavy ". Metaphorical comparisons are notoriously seductive : they tempt fancy to riot and dazzle good sense into illusion.

The history of the word " wit " is a record of a degeneration in meaning. From mental insight to the nimbler, quicker, more picturesque apprehensions, and from these to mere lively or truculent plays of fancy—so the story runs. A survey of this history from Bacon till now discloses this process of transition. Two features run clearly through the historical sequence in the estimates of wit : the identification of the witticism with the revelation of likeness between dissimilars and its inclusion among the varieties of the ludicrous. This descent of the word " wit " did not take place down a straight, continuous slope, any more than it is now uniformly degraded to trivial occasions. Various meanings lingered together, as they linger together now. But there is a general course discernible in its history whose analysis indicates both that wit, as such, is not a variety of the ludicrous and why the witticism and the joke have been naturally, though unfortunately, confounded.

Hobbes noted in " natural wit ", which is

" gotten by use only and experience ", a
" swift succession of one thought to another ;
and steady direction to some approved end " :
wit is prompt, nimble, and directed to achievement. " Observing similitudes " is " good
wit " : a witticism detects an analogy or
likeness. It is unsteady, and inclines to the
great fancy that is one kind of madness if
" good judgment ", which observes " dis-
similitudes ", does not balance it [197]. Wit
in short, pounces on resemblances, and its
indiscriminate pouncing requires the disciplinary scrutiny of judgment.

Since men laugh at mischances and in-
decencies when there is neither wit nor jest,
Hobbes distinguished between laughters with
and without a sense of the ludicrous. Wit
and jest are here distinguished, and if men
laugh at jests that elegantly discover, *in their
wit*, absurdities in another, wit seems to beget
the jest, not to be it [198]. Desire for power
stimulates wit which varies as the source of
power is sought in riches, knowledge, or
honour [199]. Wit, Hobbes apparently thinks,
can touch the sense of power by inciting
laughter of self-applause and it can procure
laughter with a sense of the ludicrous. Wit, on
Hobbes' version, is quick, nimble, perceptive,
and inventive power that tends to be volatile
and to pounce on resemblances. It also
serves the sense of the ludicrous by begetting
jests.

Locke emphasized the same contrast as Hobbes between the volatile inventiveness of wit and the more sober restraint of judgment : ". . . wit lying most in the assemblage of ideas, and putting them together with quickness and variety wherein can be found any resemblance or congruity. . . . Judgment, on the contrary, lies quite on the other side, in separating carefully one from another ideas wherein can be found the least difference, thereby to avoid being misled by similitude and by affinity to take one thing for another ". Wit, as with Hobbes, is prompt (Locke associates " a great deal of wit and prompt memory "), always pouncing on resemblances, and thus requires the discipline of analytical judgment. Wit constructs " pleasant pictures ", its " entertainment and pleasantry " appeal to fancy, and " its beauty appears at first sight." " It also tempts the mind to rest ", " satisfied with the agreeableness of the picture and the gaiety of fancy " [200]. Hazlitt's approval of the comment by " Harris, the author of *Hermes* ", that on Locke's analysis Euclid's *Elements* would be " a collection of epigrams ", assumes that Locke was defining the ludicrous, or ludicrous wit [201]. But Locke did not identify the witticism with the laughable or ludicrous, though he recognized that it could procure amusement. In both Hobbes and Locke the essence of wit is a quick pounce on a

similarity. In the period of these two philosophers, the seventeenth century, wit was
essentially regarded as sharp capturing of
similarities with a penchant for riot that
required disciplining by the more deliberate,
scrutinizing distinctions of judgment. It also
tended to beget amused laughter with its
characteristic sense of the ludicrous.

Hobbes and Locke completed a distinction
between wit and judgment previously
immanent in Bacon. For Bacon, wit was
general inventive capacity : he commends
Queen Elizabeth for " her inventing wit in
contriving plots and overturns " in " so
dangerous times, when wits are so cun-
ning " [202]. Wit, which is " able to hold all
arguments ", is more froward, desultory, and
sportive than judgment, which is more
forward " in discerning what is true ".
Hobbes, and Locke after him, more explicitly
trace the greater irresponsibility of wit to
its hankering after " similitudes ". In privi-
leging some serious matters from the jest
Bacon observes : " There be some that think
their wits have been asleep except they dart
out somewhat that is piquant and to the
quick ". He also warns the man " that hath
a satirical vein, as he maketh others afraid
of his wit, so he had need be afraid of other's
memory " [203]. Thus Bacon observed in wit
a devotion of its ingenuity to procuring jests
and also, it may be noted, to belligerency.

In the literary tradition of the seventeenth century wit retained its sense of general mental capacity, with a stress on inventiveness, and carried an emphatic implication of effective literary expression. Dryden's " great wits " who were " to madness near allied "[204] were writers of genius. Pope's well known lines :

" True wit is nature to advantage dress'd
What oft was thought, but ne'er so well expressed "[205],

prolong into the eighteenth century the general notion of wit as effective expression. Speaking of Johnson, the great literary figure of the middle eighteenth century, Sir Walter Raleigh remarks : " in our author's time wit was the general term for intellectual powers "[206]. Johnson does think " Pope's account of wit is undoubtedly erroneous " because he " reduces it from strength of thought to happiness of language ". But, " more rigorously and philosophically considered ", wit is a " strength of thought " which contains " a combination of dissimilar images, or discovery of occult resemblances in things apparently unlike "[207]. The analysis of Hobbes and Locke is steadily pressing on the notion of wit to specialize it into a revealer of comparisons. But it is not yet distinctly degraded to purveying entertainment nor reduced to a species of the laughable. It has been freely devoted, as the names of Dryden and Pope forcibly remind us, to satirical attack.

As the eighteenth century drew to its close Burke still depended on this analysis. Since " the mind of man has naturally a far greater alacrity and satisfaction in tracing resemblances than in searching for differences ", it is natural for " a perfect union of wit and judgment " to be " one of the rarest things in the world " [208]. Wit is still the volatile disturber of judgment, excitedly hunting after comparisons, rejoicing in their disclosure, and not yet identified with a species of the ludicrous. The philosopher Reid, who was of Burke's age, observes that " one great branch of what we call wit, which, when innocent, gives pleasure to every good-natured man, consists in discovering unexpected agreements in things. The author of *Hudibras* could discern a property common to the morning and a boiled lobster—that both turned from black to red " [209]. This implies an extended mental capacity for wit, refers a devotion of one " branch " of it to pouncing on similarities, recognizes in it a source of the ludicrous, and senses its tendency, for it may not be " innocent ", to belligerency.

In the early nineteenth century Coleridge continues this distinction within wit. The detection of " identity in dissimilar things ", which is steadily assigned as the province of wit, divides into " scientific wit ", whose object, " consciously entertained, is truth ", and wit, whose object is " amusement ".

A higher name is usually reserved for " scientific wit ". " Wit " is thus being reserved for amusing comparisons, though " amusement " is probably to be construed more widely than ludicrousness. Shakespeare's wit, he adds, is fanciful, placing images in unusual connections ; " wit was the stuff and substance of Fuller's intellect ". Coleridge also distinguishes Shakespeare's wit, which pleases by surprise, from his fancy, which, in addition, leaves a gratifying image with us, and suggests that " the greater part of what passes for wit in Shakespeare " is " most exquisite humour ". Fuller's wit, he also thinks, " defrauded him of his due praise for the practical wisdom of his thoughts " and for " the beauty and variety " of his truths [210]. The status of wit is being steadily lowered to a purveyor of entertainment ; it still has an eye for similitude with another eye to the ludicrous, though it is not yet identified as a species of the laughable.

A description of wit collated from Sydney Smith, a contemporary of Coleridge, would run : a discovery of a surprising and unusual relation between ideas that has neither utility nor beauty and excites a sense of superior intelligence [211]. It is expressly restricted to the lighter side of mental activity: in Rochefoucauld's " hypocrisy is the homage which vice renders to virtue " the mere wit of the image is swallowed up in justice and value. When Sydney Smith wrote : " show a child of six years old . . . that by pressing the spring of a repeating watch you make the watch strike, and you probably raise a feeling in the child's mind precisely similar to that of wit ", he seems to retain in wit a relic of achieving power and to dissociate it from any necessary connection with the ludicrous. Wit is apparently closely connected with laughter if laughter is not so long and loud in wit as it is in humour, but, since " in a piece of wit there is but a single flash of surprise and pleasure " and the " admiration " extorted by a witticism is not " favourable to laughter ", he probably does not think of wit as actually a species of the ludicrous [212]. Similitude is replaced by the wider term " relation "; the witticism is virtually restricted to the revelation of trivial relations ; and it is observed to have a close connection with the laughable.

Hazlitt, contemporaneously with Sydney Smith and Coleridge in the earlier nineteenth century, depressed the status of wit, which " hovers round the borders of the light and trifling ". Its " favourite employment " is " to add littleness to littleness, and heap contempt on insignificance by all the arts of petty and incessant warfare." When it " describes the serious seriously, it ceases to be wit ". Since " wit, or ludicrous invention produces its effect oftenest by comparison but not always " and " frequently effects its purposes by unexpected and subtle distinctions ", Hazlitt extends the province of wit beyond comparison, as Sydney Smith does, and connects it, quite clearly, with the ludicrous. There is explicit inclusion of wit as a begetter of amusement : wit " is, in fact, a voluntary act of the mind, or exercise of invention, showing the absurd and ludicrous consciously, whether in ourselves or another." He does not, however, tumble wit completely from its higher estate, for he admits, in addition to its usual predilection for warfare, " a wit of sense and observation which consists in the acute illustration of good sense and practical wisdom by means of some far - fetched conceit or quaint imagery " [213].

Hazlitt seems to consider wit essentially as a species of the ludicrous, and Leigh Hunt, in 1846, definitely included wit and humour as two species of the laughable, which implies the ludicrous, though laughter, he suggests, need not result from everything witty or humorous [214].

Ten years after, George Eliot seems to think of wit and humour as two species of the genus laughable, though they have different natures. Humour, with its less demand on mental ripeness, is the earlier growth, and has more affinity with poetic tendencies. It has been progressively humanized from triumphant laughter and coarse practical joking into the " sympathetic presentation of incongruous elements in nature and life ". Its nature is more prolix than the " direct and irresistible force of wit ". Wit remains more cruel and coarse ; it " seizes on unexpected and complex relations ", while humour " draws its materials from situations and characteristics ". " Wit is brief, sudden, detects unsuspected analogies, and suggests confounding inferences : its closer connection with logic makes kinship between the witticism and the subtle exposure, by reasoning, of a fallacy or absurdity " [215].

The tradition of mental power lingers in this estimate of wit ; the witticism apprehends nimbly and expresses decisively ; wit reveals relations and, true to tradition, has a special pounce for similitudes. Wit is also the sword of satire, and it is by nature laughable.

For Meredith wit was more war-like laughter, like the wit of Hoyden, comic laughter being the chastizer of folly without wounds, and humour the laughing comforter of susceptibilities [216].

Towards the end of the nineteenth century, Sully, apparently, contemplates no exclusion of wit from the species of laughter at the ludicrous [217], and, in the opening of the twentieth century, Bergson distinguishes the comical word which makes us laugh at the speaker from the witty which makes us laugh at ourselves or at a third party : wit is definitely adopted, it would seem, as a species of the ludicrous. In a restricted sense wit dashes off a comic scene in a few strokes [218].

In our own day Mr Eastman applies the terms "absurdity", "comic", "wit", and "joke" to the "practical kind of humour", and apparently regards the witticism as an intellectual joke [219]. Professor McDougall seems to regard the witticism as a subtle and effective presentment of the ludicrous [220].

Freud receives the impression from a survey of continental literature that wit can be successfully studied only as part of the comic [221]. The gradual and decisive assimilation of the witticism to the joke that runs clearly through English literature is, therefore, no freak nor perversity of thought. French and German discussion of wit has been in contact with English thought, but the lines have been sufficiently distinct and sufficiently determined by their own traditions to provide a convergence from different centres upon a common recognition that wit is closely connected with the ludicrous. This close connection is as significant as it has often been deceptive. It is significant because it discloses special qualifications in wit for evoking the ludicrous, and it is often deceptive because, as if a joker were identified with his joke, wit has been mistaken for a variety of the ludicrous.

Many writers realize that amusement tends to wane as wit mounts higher. This realization is apparent in Sydney Smith's verdict on Rochefoucauld's epigram, in his judgment that the admiration extorted by wit does not favour laughter, in the dissipation of wit (the laughable) by seriousness noted by Hazlitt and in the submerging of the ludicrous element by other pleasing factors when the witticism is subtle, as McDougall observes [222]. This intimation by wit, as it turns its more serious face, that it only partners easily with the ludicrous, is misunderstood when wit is restricted to its more trivial and more aggressive forms. This restriction of wit and the reservation of other terms, such as " aphorism ", to describe the more elevated achievements of insight and expression are probably connected with the persistent haunting of more trivial wit by the ludicrous. Amused laughter may be an integral and essential part of æsthetic emotion [223], it may be an indispensable part of human life, but, when comic laughter clings too persistently to anything, it tends, because relaxation belongs to its essence, to lower that thing's prestige. The prestige of wit may have suffered through its close association with the ludicrous and this reduction of dignity been marked by a withdrawal from wit of its claim on the higher forms of insight and expression. If the concentrated expression of the higher wisdom of life is allowed to wit, the separable-ness of the witticism and the joke is at once suspected, if not obvious.

If appropriate incongruity excites the sense of the ludicrous, the predilection of the witticism for remote identities, so insisted upon by the older English writers and still insisted upon by many, should have prevented the identification of wit with the comic. The reference of the ludicrous to incongruity has wavered, however, before the wreath of laughter round flashing wit. But these older writers also perceived another characteristic feature of wit that explains its connection with laughter without requiring an identification of the two.

" Brevity is the soul of wit " : all, says Freud, speaking more particularly of French and German writers, agree on this. " The direct and irresistible force of wit ", agrees George Eliot, is brief and sudden. Like a lightning artist who portrays in a few strokes, wit concentrates a truth in a few words or a mass of truth into a moment of vivid illumination. It penetrates by epitome, as Macbeth summarized Duncan in " after life's fitful fever, he sleeps well ". It illumines by a simile, as in the Elizabethan Sir Walter Raleigh's " it is opinion, not truth, that travelleth the world without passport ". It triumphs with a dagger-thrust, like the cruel reply to Pope that an interrogation mark is a little crooked thing which asks questions.

The decisiveness of wit, its brilliant moment of achievement, presents laughter with opportunity, for the stir of its passage leaves behind that original source and necessary condition of all laughing—relief.

As many laughters can spring from a centre of physical relief, or of relief in a situation that occurs in active life, so the more purely mental relief precipitated by wit is prolific in varieties of laughter. The mental recapitulation, or simulacrum, of a physical situation in relief sequent to wit must not be too peremptorily squeezed into an analogy. An analogue of the sheer laughter of relief arising from the sudden withdrawal of menace or the sudden success of an effort can be sought in sheer laughter of witty success but not necessarily found. If an irresistible witticism seems to leave nothing unsaid, and all great or effective utterance produces a momentary impression of final and complete revelation, it may thrill with a feeling of suddenly completed satisfaction that laughs with a sheer emotion of witty achievement. A hostile witticism is a surer analogue of a final sword-thrust, for wit can result in triumphant laughter, as the vindictive practical joke or the fall of an enemy in battle can result in it. The witty exposure of a futile menace may provoke laughter and suffuse it with scorn ; contemptuous laughter may roar loudly when a witticism disrobes dignity as if a hand had plucked a man naked. These and other laughters can be stirred by wit, as they can be stirred by situations in which active life drops into relief. Thus wit can easily fall into bad odour, since its efficiency, which is part of its nature, invites its use as a sword. Addison would have nothing ill said of wit, and conceived it majestically in his allegorical description : the God of Wit, " who bore several quivers on his shoulders, and grasped several arrows in his hand ", because " there was something so amiable and yet so piercing in his looks " filled the beholder " with love and terror " [224]. But, if wit is essentially an achievement of insight and expression, it can serve scurrilous uses and may serve, as Freud insists, to indulge hostility or to secure obscene satisfaction or to rebel against authority [225]. Since the relief in the wake of wit can be so prolific in laughters, it was easy to confuse wit with a species of the laughable and to accuse it, with George Eliot, of lingering among the coarser and more cruel forms of laughter.

Since wit, though the incongruous is not its own sphere, exposes incongruities as an indirect consequence of its own proper action, it can stir the sense of the ludicrous by lodging incongruity in a situation of relief. Traill saw clearly that, when wit reveals an un- suspected similarity between two things, it

LAUGHTER AND WIT

will also display an incongruity between them.
If two things are suddenly convicted of a
concealed resemblance, they will, because their
likeness required discovery, also appear as an
ill-assorted pair. The late Henry James was
a meticulous analyst and nice in his choice of
expression. Excessive nicety and superfluity
of analysis is the bane of scrupulosity. He
was wittily compared, in his moments of super-
exactness, to a hippopotamus trying to pick
up a pea. This comparison effectively expresses an excess of analysis. As such,
supposing the criticism to be just, it is true
and perceptive, and laughter immediately
provoked by the witticism will express a
gratification following the relief of achievement. So far as a sense of the ludicrous is
aroused it is incited by the incongruous
association of a respectable and able novelist
with a clumsy amphibian. Traill, by his
sharpened sense of the function of the simile
that made it the sole method of wit, saw very
distinctly that laughter (amused laughter)
often accompanies wit because incongruity is
simultaneously displayed with the revelation
of similarity [226]. He sees that wit and laughter
of amusement have been mistaken for members
of the same family because they are such close
neighbours, and, perhaps it might be added,
such cronies. But wit is neighbourly with
all the laughters, and if a witticism is not
accompanied by comic or humorous laughter

it may be, and often is, accompanied by one of their less genial fellows.

Perhaps Hobbes thought as Traill thought, many years after, when he spoke of jests elegantly discovering, *in their wit*, absurdities in others. Reid might have nodded assent to Traill's doctrine. Many writers almost seem to imply Traill's connection between wit and humour, and only somewhat inadvertently to identify wit with an inherently laughable species. It may have been so with Hazlitt if wit is, as he says, an " exercise of invention, showing the absurd and ludicrous con- sciously. . . ." Wit *showing* the ludicrous is not far from the argument of this chapter.

Wit is a quick, vivid illumination of a truth. It may bestow its energies on trifles or exercise them on higher matters. Since relief, because the rush of wit is so vigorous and its success so striking, follows in its wake, laughters can spring up round it. Other names are often preferred for the higher reaches of wit, because its nimbleness tends to the sportive, because it tends to lose prestige by prompting laughters so readily, and because it is so ready a weapon for satire and all kinds of rebellion. It prospers largely on the metaphor, and this prosperity is one root of its loss of reputation, since metaphors are good servants who easily become riotous masters. The emphatic relief it confers is another root, for it helps it to that association with laughter which has so influenced its fortunes. Every relief-situation has a descending incongruity for its sides, and the stroke of wit indirectly manufactures incongruities or displays them. Thus the witticism tends to be, in effect, a joke and to stir a sense of the ludicrous. Wit, however, is not laughable *per se*, though it is an effective cause of the laughable.

This is no complete analysis of comic wit or of any wit. Relief and incongruity, a contrast that administers a psychical shock, are always present in the ludicrous, but they do not compass the full richness of the comical or the humorous. So with wit : " Any one better apprehends what it is by acquaintance than I can inform him by description. It is indeed a thing so versatile and multiform . . . that it seemeth no less hard to make a portrait of Proteus, or to define the figure of the fleeting air " [227].

CHAPTER X

ACCORDING to a now common notion, of modern origin, we laugh, as Falstaff was a coward, on instinct. This notion is natural to an age which looks for function and, in studying anything, thinks first of its use or purpose. Instinct is too purposeful and theorists are too anxious for laughing to be useful for laughter not to be claimed as an instinct. Laughter is still approached in different ways, and, in particular, is still studied from an æsthetic standpoint. But the psychological and sociological approach, so prominent in present thought, is so thoroughly preoccupied with instincts that it is almost predestined to include laughter among them. Some writers who hesitate to make laughter, and comic or humorous laughter in particular, a member of the same company as anger, fear, and other instincts, draw it as closely as they can to this company. When thought centres on usefulness, when purposeful instincts stand in the foreground of thought and when pervasive, perplexing laughter taunts its would-be interpreters with their failures, the attempt to solve the problem of laughter by treating it as an instinct amenable to the principles applicable to instincts is virtually inevitable. This attempt is one prominent characteristic of thinking to-day.

If we were amused as feeling or thinking statues, if they could exist, would be amused ; if the sense of the ludicrous suffused our minds without even a ripple on our bodies ; if we did not smile or grin or guffaw or contort our bodies when we are pleased or amused or triumphant or elated, there might be no talk of instinctive laughter. There *is* such talk, and, at the moment, plenty of it, because we do smile and grin and guffaw and sometimes very vigorously exercise our bodies in hearty laughing. The familiar, peculiar, and emphatic " mechanical motion " of laughter naturally provokes a comparison with flight stirred by fear or attack urged by anger. Instincts have an emotional side and an active, physically manifest side. The emotion of fear can be read on the flight of a frightened child. If the motions of escape are instinctive, or part of an instinct, the " happy convulsion " of laughter may be instinctive too, for amusement can be read on a laugh, as anger can be read on a blow.

The response of theorists to the suggestion that laughter is an instinct has been sensitized by the influence of behaviouristic psychology. Naturalists watch the actions of animals and they can observe a small bird's dash for safety when a hawk hovers, as we can observe a cloud hurry across a windy sky. The psychologist can study his own consciousness, or, at any rate what he has been accustomed to call his own consciousness. He can note his own joy, his own pain when he loses a tooth to the forceps, his recollection of his past, his "mental image" or mental picture, as he has been accustomed to consider it, of the past scene which he recollects, and he can note both his thinking and his thoughts. He cannot watch his neighbour's thoughts or inspect his emotions, but he can watch his actions. The naturalist spontaneously assumes a feeling of fear in the fleeing bird, and the psychologist, with equal spontaneity, assumes that the little girl in the next garden feels fear when she shrinks from a dog. Now it is easier to watch the actions of a lobster than to know how it feels or thinks. Human actions, even, are more obvious to the observer than human emotions or thoughts. The conscious part of human life seems to be known through its physically active part, which includes speaking and writing, and since we are often uncertain about people's motives and frequently misunderstand their intentions, thoughts, or feelings, mental life seems to be somewhat precariously surmised from behaviour. Watch the bird flee, then, as you would watch the flow of its blood through a microscope, experience seems to enjoin, and watch your neighbours as you watch their motor-cars—without reck of " mental images " or anything else mental and privately concealed for us to surmise in their bodies and actions. This behaviouristic method of studying perceptible actions and ignoring mental processes or states of consciousness appears the more profitable because careful study reveals a great sensitiveness in the body to mental states.

A slight pin-prick, or the threat of one, sends an electric current over the palm of the hand, and if a sensitive galvanometer, indicating the passage of electric currents by the movements of a spot of light, is connected with the patient's palm the occurrence and intensities of emotions in him are indicated by the spot's movements and their range [228]. When the travelling spot of light adds, as it were, to the gestures of the body, indicating emotion as the excited dance of a child indicates it, study is naturally attracted by this and similar extensions of possibility in studying human behaviour. The physiologist can trace the effect of expecting food in a preparation of the body for digestion—saliva waters the hungry man's mouth as he sits down to eat. He can detect an increase of sugar in the blood after anxiety or pain or fear or strain, discover a physiological record in the body of excitement from mixing with a crowd or listening to music, and read hunger in the contractions of an alimentary canal [229]. A simple experiment opens to inspection a wide range of actions that are more subdued than obvious gestures or movements. The experimenter suspends a gold ring by a silk thread in an empty glass and concentrates his thoughts on the hour of day. Presently the tinkling of the hour on the glass announces slight bodily motions corresponding to the thought [230]. Scientific ingenuity has assiduously added to our knowledge of human behaviour, by many methods analogous to these, many subtler responses to thought and feeling.

The psychological laboratory and the resources of physiology have so increased the possibilities of studying mind, or consciousness, through behaviour or bodily processes that extreme behaviourists say it should be studied only thus. Thus Thorndike says that a man's anxiety or toothache can be observed in his actions in exactly the same physical way that the temperature of his body can be taken by a thermometer [231]. Still more absolute behaviourists affirm that we study men's minds by thoroughly observing their gestures, all the overt and subdued motions, external and internal, of their bodies, and the chemical changes in their organisms, because there is nothing more to study. Thus Professor Watson refuses to use the word " consciousness ", and defines psychology as " that division of natural science which takes human activity and conduct as its subject matter "[232]. If this and other absolute behaviourist utterances are taken literally, and they seem to be intended literally, they mean that if you observe every motion of and in the body of a man and every chemical change in it, you know the *whole* man. They mean also that a complete cinematograph picture of a man's laugh, including every motion and change occurring in his body, would be laughter. But his sense of the ludicrous, his amusement, if he laughed at a joke, would be omitted by the cinema. The audience would sympathetically insert it because they have themselves laughed amusedly. To spectators who had never experienced the " sudden glory " of amused laughter, who were strangers to ludicrous emotion, the cinema would portray a curious, enigmatical contortion of a human body, not a fit of laughing. This extreme behaviouristic insistence on the body overemphasizes the reasonable behaviouristic determination to consider the whole psycho-physical organism, mind and body together. The emotion of fear is more intelligible when the motions of flight are observed to remove the body from real or fancied danger, and it is natural to look for light on laughter in its physical expression. The mechanics and physiology of laughter disclose very clearly, as previously noted, the element of relaxation through interrupted effort, of relief, in laughing. The older theorists were less behaviouristic and more exclusively devoted to the mental aspect of laughter than the modern. This did not prevent them from suggesting for laughter or even from anticipating Professor McDougall. "I make haste to laugh", said Beaumarchais, "for fear of being obliged to weep" [233]. McDougall's estimate of laughter as an instinct devoted to suppressing unnecessary sympathy elaborates into a complete theory the aptness of some misfortunes, noted by Hazlitt, to "afford us amusement from the very rejection of their false claims upon our sympathy" [234]. McDougall recognizes both the conscious and physical aspects of laughter, and there seems to be no express behaviouristic identification of laughing with a purely physical and physiological disturbance of the body, though Watson implies it; but the modern attention to the physical aspects of mental life, particularly in connection with instincts, has doubtless been very influential on the modern estimate of laughter as an instinct.

"Laughter", wrote Mandeville, "is a mechanical motion, which we are naturally *thrown into* when we are unaccountably pleased" [235]. The hunting wasp, Sphex, is "naturally thrown into" a complicated "mechanical motion" when she paralyses crickets by stinging them thrice—in the neck, between the joint of a front thoracic segment, and towards the abdomen—and devotes them, suspended between life and death, to the jaws of her future offspring by laying her eggs on them.[236]. The skilled surgery of the wasp, which pierces the effective nervous centres of the cricket and adjusts its venomous attack to produce a perfectly immobile suspended animation without death so that the grub may have fresh meat without danger from the victim's struggles, is spontaneously exerted without training. The performance anticipates without the wasp being anticipatory, for a larder is stocked for future grubs by a mother who, since she dies before they break from the eggs, can scarcely understand what she does or why she does it. Aristotle speaks of " natural desires ", such as those for food or sexual love, " of which the body is a necessary instrument " and which do " not spring from a definite theory "[237]. If we neglect " desire " for the obvious performances of laughter and the wasp, we observe in each both an operation by body and an independence of " definite theory ". Both suggest automatism ; both appear as bits of routine predestined by the constitution of the organism to occur during life ; both seem to be performances into which the organism is *thrown* by circumstances.

Both the spontaneous, unreflectingly automatic interjection of the laugh and the hunt similarly interjected into the life of the wasp seem to be, in terms of Bergson's familiar note on instinct, extensions into behaviour, into the overt bodily actions constituting activity in the arena of life, of the unreflecting, spontaneous, apparently automatic physiological processes within the body. We laugh and Sphex hunts much as we breathe or as our hearts beat. The laughing and the hunting are more occasional than breathing, but they appear, when their moments come, to be equally predestined in life's routine.

Laughter so strongly suggests an action that the body is *set* to perform when appropriate occasions touch off the setting that *The New English Dictionary* deliberately defines the laugh as the *instinctive* expression of mirth or the sense of the ludicrous. It also, as appears from the continued course of its definition, suspects its instinctive character from the power of certain sensations, notably tickling, to occasion it. Though laughter, which does nothing but agitate the stationary body and " while it lasts, slackens and unbraces the mind, weakens the faculties, and causes a kind of remissness and dissolution in the powers of the soul " [288], cannot be the established response to tickling, which makes the body struggle and requires tension instead of relaxation, the easy access to stimulation of laughter enjoyed by tickling and other sensations marks a human readiness to be thrown into laughing. The " happy convulsion " is so nicely prepared, so frequently incited, in the human frame, and so promptly precipitated by its occasions, that the insistence on its instinctive character by many modern writers is wholly intelligible.

Laughter confirms the verdict on its instinctiveness by appearing as an innate, indurated tendency, common to all members of the human race, to act in a definite way on certain occasions that has not to be learned, though it may be stimulated by the laughter of others and require some practice before it settles into an easily running and readily provoked habit. To the extent that the infant seems to be born to acquire the habit of laughing inevitably, laughter seems to be instinctive. If it were only qualified to laugh in the sense that it is only qualified to learn the *ABC*, assuming the habit only if it happens to be a habit enjoined by its social circle and laughing only because those around it laugh, the verdict might be doubted. But, even though Lilly meant that North American Indians and Cingalese Veddas do not laugh when he said they had no sense of the ludicrous [259] and said rightly, laughter is too constant among variations of human habit for its instinctiveness to be suspected because it appears to be at all sporadic. Human beings seem as naturally inclined to laugh as to run when they are frightened, so that flight from danger and laughter appear to be equally instinctive.

Unhesitatingly accepted instincts, like the behaviours of fear and anger, usually extend their ancestry well below man into the animal world. Flight from danger and assault roused by insult or frustration, as when a cornered animal, because it cannot escape, converts retreat into attack, are obvious in animals, though their *feelings* of fear or anger are surmised. Laughter is obviously younger historically than either of those ancient instincts—fear and anger. It did not flourish, whether as an instinct or not, until man adopted it, for, even if apes laugh and jackdaws relish practical jokes with a tinge of the amusement destined to pervade human laughter, both the physical act of laughing and the characteristic sense of the ludicrous have a relatively languishing existence among animals. Fear is as characteristic of animals as it is of men ; animal laughter or joking is little more than a hint of human laughter. Even if dogs do occasionally show a sense of humour [240], laughter is admittedly a young instinct.

The youth of laughter may be pertinent to its nature and require attention from the theorist. Whatever significance the predominantly human origin of laughter may have, or not have, laughing is unique among the instincts, if it is one of them. Unhesitatingly accepted instincts have unhesitatingly discerned uses. No one can mistake the purposefulness of fear and anger. The absence of body that is better than presence of mind when danger lurks is obviously secured by the flight of fear. The soldier, who, during the battle, crouched where the bullets were thickest—in the ammunition waggon—knew why nature had endowed him with fear. Anger, as obviously, warns off the assailant or precipitates that counter-attack which, according to military axiom, is the best defence. The purpose of fear is not obscured, though its defeat is desired, when it is laid under discipline. Military drill, by its very measures to keep soldiers firm before danger, recognizes the function of their fear-instincts. When the mild answer is found to assuage wrath and advised as a surer defence than anger, the original purpose of anger is still evident. The tendency of all emotional instincts to defeat their own purposes by excessive violence or inopportune intervention, as when anger makes a boxer hit too wildly to land his blows or fear haps on a second danger by fleeing from a first that would collapse if faced, does not dissociate them from these purposes. The flight of fear and the counter-attack of anger, though their purposes may be better served, either wholly or on occasion, by other methods or defeated by excess of emotion or violence, have an obviously discernible function, and, in general, the more clearly behaviour is instinctive, the more clearly it is purposeful. When an instinct persists in acting in a wrong situation, like Fabre's processionary caterpillars circling endlessly round the moulding on a palm vase [241], it advertizes its purpose by its very determination to serve it under all circumstances. Now no specific purpose *seems* to be appropriated to laughter. " Seems " should be used advisedly, for the mistaken attempts to appropriate a definite purpose to laughter, in according it instinctive status, may simply have failed to observe its real function. But, since these appropriations differ in different writers, the instinctive function of laughter is clearly less obvious than the functions of fear or anger. Since an instinct frequently in action has a defined purpose laughter is unique, if it is an instinct, by being both frequently in action and enigmatic.

Mr Eastman does not observe with enough care the uniqueness of the " mechanical motion " of laughter, and does not realize fully the ambiguity of calling it an " act ". Laughter in a wide sense *is* " a part of what we do ", but he is too convinced that it is not " merely something that happens when we have ceased to do anything " when he insists that it " is an act . . . a fulfilment in its own proper degree of the social instinct " [242]. The laugher *does* nothing to anyone or anything other than himself. He does nothing even to himself in the sense that a frightened man moves himself from a dangerous spot. Professor McDougall sees more clearly : " the instinct to laugh is peculiar in that its impulse seeks to effect no change in the relation of organisms to the outer world, but terminates in, and finds its satisfaction in, the bodily changes produced by laughter " [243]. Laughter is not an *act* as a blow is an angry act or flight is a fearful act. Neither is it, properly speaking, an " act of acceptance " [244]. The laugher simply holds his sides and laughs—his laughter is an *action broken*.

The child smiles, according to Eastman, in acceptance of his social circle, and from that " smile of dawning laughter " all its smiles and laughter grow. His smile is part of his gregarious instinct, his instinct to welcome, join, and act with his companions, and his laughter is developed through play, itself " in its elementary form instinctive ". This instinct to smile and laugh in joyful acceptance of comradeship in play " is the germ and simple rudiment of what we call the sense of humour ". The new, unique feeling of amusement, that humorous emotion which is unique and unanalysable into more simple components, the latest instinct to evolve, is "an act of welcoming a playful shock or disappointment ". The giggle, with its tinge of amusement, evolves from " the smile of gratification which greets a friendly look " to ripen into the laugh enamoured of the joke which is "created by the exact coincidence of a playful shock or disappointment with a playful or genuine satisfaction ". Since tickling is the most crude and elementary form of play and humorous emotion often suffuses the laughter of the tickle, nursery tickling is an authentic and first picture of humour [245].

Thus, according to Eastman, the laugh is essentially laughter of greeting flourishing in an atmosphere of play. Companions are greeted first with a smile, and then, as humorous laughter begins in the giggle, the ludicrous receives its greeting. The laugh is the ripened product of this double greeting to companionship and the amusing.

Disciplinary laughter is more like rejection than acceptance, and Meredith, for whom "folly is the natural prey of the comic " [246], aligns himself, as Eastman himself expresses it, to laughter fundamentally as an act of rejection. The descent of ridicule upon folly or Meredith's non-contemptuous silvery laughter at human foolishness can be ingeniously estimated as greeting or acceptance of absurdity. Laughter, humorous laughter, Eastman would doubtless say, greets the ludicrous in folly, and contempt, if contempt is present, attends laughter without being part of it. But Sir Thomas Browne would with difficulty descry pure acceptance in the laugh of " the severe schools " by which he refused to be dislodged from the " philosophy of Hermes ", and an act of greeting is invaded with surprising ease by scorn and rejection if Eastman is right. If theorists still incline so persistently to include a residual sense of superiority in all laughter, animus, though restricted, must linger pertinaciously in the laugh. The prevalence of derision-theories of laughter in the past and the persistent reluctance to exclude the stroke of superiority from laughing intimate plainly how animus has haunted the laugh. This haunting by animus of what is essentially a genial greeting, and an instinctive greeting at that, might be conjecturally explained, but it suggests that a more catholic version of laughing, opening it more freely to the triumph, scorn, self-congratulation, and, it must not be forgotten, to the sympathy, that undoubtedly freely enter it, should replace its identification with an act of acceptance.

If laughing is a breaking-off, an interrupted action expending its superfluity on the body, it is a special act and appropriate to a variety of situations. It is special because its function is to break, or express a break in, other actions that specifically relate the laugher to his surroundings, as the children laughed when they had run from Washington Irving. It fits many occasions because it interrupts so many different actions : the struggle of battle, the response to a threat quickly judged to be futile, the suddenly successful effort. It can express acceptance and it can express rejection. Different feelings or emotions collect round it because it can break off triumphantly or scornfully or, in some purely mental situations, amusedly, or in a variety of other ways.

McDougall enumerates the constituents of instinct thus : it is a psycho-physical disposition ; it determines a perception of and attention to certain objects ; it contains a specific impulse to specific action ; and it is attended by a *specific emotional excitement* [247]. Each instinct has a characteristic primary impulse and a specific emotion [248]. Eastman, who defers to McDougall's account of instinct, has provided laughter with a specific action, acceptance ; but he has, apparently, also provided it with two emotions. " The smile of gratification which greets a friendly look " is the laughter of greeting, in being or in embryo, and he distinguishes it from the subsequent and unique feeling of amusement [249]. The instinct of laughter has thus at least two emotional accompaniments — gratification and amusement. McDougall himself, more consistently, attaches the single emotion of

" amusement " to laughter. He also makes laughter more emphatically purposeful than Eastman. Even if laughter is not vague in its role as a special instinct of acceptance, it smacks of the superfluous. An instinct devoted to stopping the excesses of sympathy has a well-defined function, even if it is a superfluous one. If there is any truth in the progressive humanization of laughter that has been affirmed in these pages laughter is more a means of letting sympathy in than of keeping it out.

Both these writers have a keener sense of the conscious accompaniments of the physical act of laughing than of that act itself, though they do insist on the instinctiveness of laughter and discuss its mechanics. Sympathy, of course, may prompt us to assist in the chase of a lost hat and laughter check the impulse because the disaster is seen to be too trifling to require our efforts. But it is, unfortunately, a doubtful reading of human history that assumes a necessity for a special instinct to restrain sympathy. There is cruelty enough in the human record to suggest that men have never had much difficulty in restraining their sympathies, without a special instinct to assist them. So pervasive an instinct as laughter, devoted to correcting sympathetic excesses, would probably delay the growth of sympathy, already with enough enemies, more than it would hinder it from destructive excesses. Laughter breaks response to false claims upon sympathy as it breaks other responses when action is called off, but it seems, so far as it is a specific action at all, to be specifically a breaking reaction and can occur, when the situation precipitated by the breaking is one of relief, in a great variety of circumstances.

If " laughter is an instinctive reaction of aberrant type ", and if " its impulse " differs from most instinctive impulses by terminating in the body of the laugher, it may be more catholic in its emotions than more normal instincts. An instinct that arrests other instincts as part of its proper function or nature, for the sudden arrest of fear or anger is apt to excite laughter, may be loose in its emotional attachments. It may be as misleading to speak uncritically of " its impulse " as to speak uncritically of its " act ", for it seems to scatter impulses gathered for other purposes rather than exercise a specific impulse of its own. As a spill-way for energy or impulse no longer needed, it is peculiar among those combinations of emotion and action that invite the name of instinct. If laughter has a specific emotion at all, sheer relief would seem to be the strongest candidate for the office. But it seems clear that it does not confine itself to one emotion any more than it confines itself to breaking off one call to action. The relief of laughter can disarm hostility as well as disable sympathy. The protean possibilities of laughter have constantly seduced theorists into choosing one of them to the exclusion of the rest. It can accept or reject, express a social welcome or suppress sympathy ; it can break struggle into triumph or the call of a futile menace into scorn ; it can discipline by ridicule or humorously link men into sympathy.

If every action into which we are inevitably thrown when the conditions are appropriate is an instinct, laughter is an instinct. If an instinct has a specific impulse, the instinctiveness of laughter is more doubtful. If every instinct has its own private emotion and one only, laughter is no instinct. "There is a real distinction", wrote Reid, "between persons within the house, and those that are without it ; yet it may be dubious to which the man belongs that stands upon the threshold"[250]. Laughter may be a troublesome threshold man—now asking for inclusion among instincts and now protesting against the inclusion. But it is more important to understand what laughter is than to arrange the definition of "instinct" to its idiosyncrasies.

Eastman says that "humorous emotion" is an instinct because it is unique, does not analyse into more simple components, and, in accordance with McDougall's first test for an instinct, is socially infectious [251]. Insistence on these criteria would multiply instincts almost to the point of indecency, and, if laughter is simply to be a member of so motley an assemblage, let it be an instinct. But it must not be assumed, because of this inclusion, that laughter in general, which need not be amused or only amused, appropriates only one emotion and serves only one specific purpose.

The " mechanical motion " of laughing is an indurated, innate habit impressed upon the human body that breaks other actions into relief. It may break the violent struggle of battle or the more subdued physical movements or tension of anticipatory attention. " The muscular actions constituting it are distinguished from most others " by being " purposeless " [252], if " purposeless " means that it interrupts the purposes of other activities. Its purpose may, however, be the interruption of the activities it breaks and, perhaps, of their purposes. This purpose, if it is conceded, is reflected in its function of spill-way for gathered energy, whose superfluity is expended on the body, and, perhaps, in the using up of " energizing secretions ", such as the extra sugar in the blood, that the interrupted effort no longer requires [253].

Secondary functions develop out of primary, and as the by-products of an industry may become more important or prominent than the original productions, become more significant than they. So laughter, originally a throwing of body (and mind) out of gear, seems, by an intimate association with the sense of the ludicrous, to have become an important contributor to the geniality of life, a check on folly, and, though it may be turned to base uses, a promoter of sane judgment.

Since the moment of arrest favours the flow of emotion, whatever is the precise connection between emotion and action, the relief of laughter seems to be naturally qualified for emotional accompaniment, and, since the fundamental situation of relief varies with the nature of the broken activity, the emotional accompaniment is likely to be variable. Many emotions appear to gather naturally round laughter and the nature of laughter seems to invite their gathering. The sense of the ludicrous is a specific emotional accompaniment of laughter in the sense that laughter is its only physical expression ; but in many laughs other emotions accompany amusement, and every laugh need not be amused, though the comic tends to tinge and pervade all varieties of laughter.

CHAPTER XI

THE FUNCTION AND ÆSTHETICS OF LAUGHTER

LAUGHTER, as Montaigne said of Aristotle, " hath an oare in every water, and medleth with all things ". Its infinite variety almost convinced Ribot that it had no single fundamental cause [254]. Now a busybody who interfered with a dozen matters in a forenoon might appear in too many different roles to seem to a casual observer to be definitely occupied. But the busybody has a single impulse to meddle, and laughter, though it would be unfairly described as a busybody, resembles him in being a confirmed meddler with a definite method of meddling. It meddles with all kinds of activities by breaking them off into relief and presenting an incongruity that stirs the sense of the ludicrous, when relaxation suddenly supervenes as effort or tension is suddenly interrupted. Thus laughter has a single source in a situation of incongruous relief and a nature as multiple as this situation is various. If " nearly all comic theorists are comic monists " and are

" altogether persuaded that laughter must have one cause and one cause only " [255], they may have sensed the ultimate singleness of all laughter. But they may have surrendered to a lazy and erroneous presupposition, for the mind loves to make many things into one, as a tidy housewife loves to pack many garments into one chest. Comic laughter, also, is more easily referred to one cause than all the varieties of laughter collectively, and, in a sense rightly, since the sense of the ludicrous seems to be specially associated with a perception of the incongruity in the general situation of incongruous relief.

The human mind, when its speculative fervour is fired, can be almost incredibly determined to compel things into singleness of aspect. The passionate *monocentrism* of much Hindu philosophy yearned so for oneness that it denied reality to any change or anything that changed. The repetition of " the mystic syllable *om* " stupefied the devotee till he forgot there was anything else in the world ; his intelligent moments were plied with a doctrine of the illusoriness of a world that deluded him till he realized its illusoriness ; his goal was a condition more remote from waking life than the fitful consciousness of dreaming sleep and more remote from it even than a sleep that is dreamless [256]. Such a regime for apprehending the oneness of reality, by making the devotee so incapable of apprehending any disturbing change that he also became unconscious of the oneness on which his soul was set, is the very ecstasy of monocentrism. Touches of this ecstasy are apt to betray the mind regularly into error.

A single formula is to the philosophical mind what monogamy is to the ethical—an ideal goal. The collection, in Frith's picture of *Derby Day*, of incidents dispersed through space and scattered through time under one view, places the mind's hand on many things as though they were one. The controlling conditions of the mind's activity predispose it to injudicious and even intemperate unification. The seductiveness of wit, the theme of such solemn warnings by Hobbes, Locke, and their successors, derives from an impulsive combination of two things into one through a remote likeness : when an illustration or a metaphor is mistaken for a real analogy unification is excessive. "Alertness of mind", the "flying abroad of all the faculties to the open doors and windows at every passing rumour", is more content with a miscellany than attention, which "is the concentration of every" faculty "in a single focus, as in the alchemist over his alembic at the moment of expected projection". Since "attention is the stuff that memory is made of", and memory is not only "accumulated genius" [257] but the sign of comprehension, for we remember most easily what we comprehend most completely, the concentrated act of attention is the method of the reflective mind. Now the act of attention is not a fixed, unswerving stare, which is hypnotic, but a steadily poised look that, as it were, revolves round its object. Its appropriate object, therefore, is many things combined into one so that it can be grasped in a single act and correspond to the variations in the attentive movement. "Marshal thy notions into a handsome method" for "things orderly fardled up under heads are most portable" [258] was Fuller's maxim for remembering, and Sydney Smith echoed many before him, as he was echoed by many after him, by observing that "memory may be wonderfully strengthened by referring single facts and observations to one simple principle" [259]. The monocentering mind, always seeking for one centre round which attention can revolve, is always attempting to convert the act of *apprehension* from an indiscriminating sweep of things into an act of *comprehension* which grasps a system of things both articulated and single. It strives to comprehend as nearly as possible in one richly filled act of attention as much as it can as singly as it can. This is its strength and its weakness : its strength because it thus strengthens and completes understanding, its weakness because hankering after " one simple prin-

ciple" sees more simply, in many instances,
than it should. Things are not necessarily
either as simple as we desire or simple in the
way we simplify them. Thus a pardonable
suspicion may linger round the universal
formula for laughter as a bodily and mental
experience characterizing a situation of incongruous relief. But it seems possible to lull it
by observing the characteristic mechanics of
laughter that provides it with a backbone,
by noting how this formula adapts itself
to all varieties of laughing, as one mathe-
matical equation expresses many different
sections of a cone by assigning different
constants to its variables, and by realizing
how the many different theories regarding
the nature and function of laughter circle
round this formula—indicating it as the centre
upon which they tend to converge. The
generality of the formula, it must also be
remembered, leaves plenty of scope for particular analyses of particular laughters. No
machine is fully explained by noting that it
does not endeavour to supply more energy than
is originally put into it and no laughter, probably, is fully explained by the general formula.
But the principle that all energy obtained from
a machine must first be supplied to it regulates
the performances of machinery and, similarly,
the occurrences of a situation containing incongruous relief regulate and determine the
nature, origin and functions of laughter.

Unless body and mind go their own ways, with no reck of each other, the mental accompaniments of laughter must be intelligibly connected with its physical expression. If the physical expression is uniform, the many laughters must conform to a fundamental plan that can be read in the act of laughter. If the act of laughing breaks off an action and expends superfluity upon the body in a squandering upon a precipitated situation of relief, the emotions, and ideas so far as they exist, of the laughter must have an intelligible connection with this characteristic and uniform situation. If laughter is always a break, as its characteristic " mechanical motion " intimates so distinctly, it will present itself in a single aspect throughout its varieties, and if it breaks in on many occasions it will differ with the situations it precipitates, for all relief is relief from something, and bare, abstract relief is less than a shadow. Relief, like most if not all else, is relative to circumstances and may be, as it were, a relative peace surrounded by storm. A frontiersman, when he came home, found his wife and children dead, scalped, and mutilated. He burst out laughing and, constantly exclaiming : " it is the funniest thing I ever heard of ", laughed on convulsively till he ruptured a blood-vessel [260]. A hair's-breadth divided this terrible laugh from a flood of tears. Warm hopes were suddenly broken and a quiescence, chill like death itself, settled on the wounded soul. A glimpse of the incongruity in the home-coming grimly engaged the sense of amusement that confirmed body and soul in a relief too despairing to weep with even a sense of the vainness of effort. Nothing could be done —tears or laughter: what did it matter? Amusement chose a wild laugh. There was relief, as in all laughter, but it was a mere violent lull in a storm that must be faced again. The wild laugh was hollow and joyless like the relief it expressed. Laughter may be terribly versatile—its relief may be hellish and its mirth joyless.

In such a devil's jest, expecting a home and finding a charnel-house, Angell might see a direful exaggeration of the disorganization always inflicted, though usually less savagely, by the joke [261]. Everything was broken for the frontiersman, and his laugh, as it destroyed his search for a house, left him nothing else to seek. The disorganization of normal laughter is more evanescent—breaking off one activity and, after temporary disablement, most marked in the prostration of hearty laughter, freeing the laughter for others. " For the laugh ", writes Greig, " is manifestly disorderly, in that it does not contribute towards the end of any behaviour of which a very young child can be supposed capable ; and it retains this character in most of the behaviour of later life. It is generally interruptory and can only be regarded as contributory when it is deliberately *used* by the laugher ", and, he adds, " the smile and the laugh are seldom more than mere flashes in behaviour "[262]. Behaviour is best judged by a systematized series of actions and not by single actions, as the course of a planet appears in its orbit and not in its momentary position. So the " behaviour-cycle ", many actions combined into one deed under one purpose or impulse, is the favourite modern unit of behaviour. A leap from bed, a hurried toilette, a quick breakfast, a rush to the station, a purchased newspaper, a sequestrated seat in the train, and a continuous sequence of further actions, major and minor, compose a total behaviour-cycle of attention to business. It is good to think in wholes if the parts are not forgotten, but preoccupation with behaviour-cycles sometimes has this forgetfulness. Holt almost suggests, if he does not nearly say, that the belated sleeper does not really jump from his bed when his rising is overdue because he is really attending to business[263]. When behaviour-cycles occupy thought, the fitfulness of laughter tends to dissipate any sense of its functions because its momentary appearances are " mere flashes in behaviour ".

The mechanics of laughter, a transparent interruption of activity, intimates a significance for these intermittent appearances.

Laughter breaks an adjustment when neither it nor any further adjustment is immediately needed : summoned energies are expended on the body because they are not required. Normally it disorganizes only by punctuating activity with relief. The laugh of triumph, after success in struggle, disorganizes fighting activity but the relief is welcome since it simply demobilizes what need no longer be mobilized. Laughter is, normally, disorganization in the sense that military demobilization is disorganization—it dispenses with preparations that have served their purpose. The situation of relief intermittently precipitated by laughter is, whether primarily or secondarily, an important element in the behaviour-cycle, for it has a similar function to the rest during the route-march. It is a moment of recuperation, a respite in the present from immediate urgency in the future, and McDougall, though he theoretically confines laughter to the one duty of correcting excess of sympathy, notes that " the bodily movements of laughter . . . bring about a condition of *euphoria* or general well-being " [264]. It would be tedious to recite the testimonials to the *euphoria* of laughter. It is true, no doubt, as Greig insists, that pleasant movements usually contribute to the smooth movement of the whole behaviour-cycle while interruptory incidents are displeasing [265] : the business man is pleased if he catches his train and interjaculatory if he misses it. But laughter is, normally, as Socrates remarked of the jest, " a *pleasant* interruption ", and it is pleasant because its interruption is relief—a relaxation from un-required effort. " The feeling of the whole behaviour " does not give the whole " key to the situation ", for pleasing laughter can suddenly break off an imminent quarrel. The general behaviour situation has its say : a situation of relief must be provided for the laugh.

The grief of " the whole behaviour ", as the melancholy of Jacques spread through all, may turn the natural joy of laughter into sadness, as the frontiersman's laughter was grievous [266], but, since relief is usually pleasurable, saddened laughter is laughter deprived of its birthright. Laughter must be given its opportunities—this must be conceded to the behaviour-cycle ; but it is a sign that an opportunity for relief has been accepted. It also seems, when it is carefully regarded, to try to make the best of its opportunities.

Many things happen in the combination of body and mind whose activities constitute human life as if a purpose presided over its own welfare and over the welfare of its community. The private welfare of human life is more pertinent to the function of laughter and more pertinent also are those occurrences in mind and body that happen with spontaneous apartness from conscious will or purpose as if prompted by a vigilant guardian spirit. If the infant were not prompted to suck, it would die ; coagulation tends to stanch the bleeding cut ; the call of danger urges to safety by flight or braces for struggle ; the finger sharply withdraws itself from the painful burn that would destroy it ; thinking is often more like something happening to us than our own act, as if actuated by a purpose to compel us to know for our own good. Now laughter acts as if it has purpose in it. It happens to us, it occurs in us as our eyes wink, and we attempt to provoke it by a jest as we strike a finger at naturally winking eyes. It makes the rest of relief doubly recuperative, multiplies its pleasure and seeks from it a maximum of benefit. The sense of the ludicrous is in the true vein of laughter, for it enriches those halts that laughter makes contributary to the enhancement of life. Comic perception does enhance life, and in this unique achievement laughter constantly acts as though it sought to convert the act of breaking off activities into its greatest profit for the laugher.

When the laugh is abnormal it acts as though it pursued its intent with mistaken zeal. Such mistaken zeal was the tragedy of the frontiersman's laugh. His amusement was laughter striving to make of relief the greatest uplift. That sense of the ludicrous, intruding on grief, was laughter, strenuous in purpose, bent on its opportunity and eager for *euphoria*, aiming at exhilaration. If the man had wept he might have lived, for tears are the natural outlet of grief. Such destructive excess of zeal marks an inherent tendency in the occurrence of laughter to exploit the situation of relief for the well-being of the laugher.

As the laugh of triumph suffuses victory with a gratified sense of achievement, so comic perception suffuses pleasant interruptions with a greater elation. Laughter, in its purposeful aspect, for it has a *purposeful* aspect whether the wise decide that it is *purposive* or not, *is* the elater of pleasant interruptiveness. It adds a " sudden glory " to the contempt of scorn as it does to the triumph of victory and, with less ungraciousness, to the ludicrously incongruous which is the incongruity of situations of relief. This sense of the ludicrous is laughter's final perseverance in aiming at elation, its favourite method of obtaining it, and its principal, if not its only, claim to æsthetic value. The " happy convulsion " of laughter begins its endeavour after the elation of pleasant interruption with a benefit to the body, and comic perception ends that endeavour with a benefit more pre-eminently bestowed upon the mind.

Laughter turns relief to greater profit. It turns a diverted action into a pleasant gymnastic and makes the body glow with an exercise snatched from the hurry of life. The act of laughing is filled with the candour of laughter's purpose. That rocking to and fro on which laughter expends the gathered energy it cuts short is an earnest of a continued effort by the laugh. The laughing body is a relieved body under genial exercise, and that genial exercise turns relief to greater profit. The sense of the ludicrous does more exclusively for the mind what laughs do more exclusively for the body : thus laughing and comic perception march together, for both further the purpose in laughter to add exhilaration to relief.

All æsthetic interests enhance life and enrich it with new values. They also withdraw themselves partially from the stir, hurry, and pressure of affairs. This element of withdrawal is the constantly repeated burden of discussions on æsthetics. Æsthetic objects, says Lord Balfour, using " æsthetic " in a wide sense, have value because they arouse *contemplative* emotions, self-contained and self-sufficient, that *subserve no purpose*[267]. They do not, that is, serve purposes that are somewhat indefinitely, though on the whole intelligibly, termed useful or practical. If beauty is a non-erroneous illusion, as Professor Alexander suggests [268], it neither invites logical protest nor requires practical participation—for illusion is no appropriate stimulus to action. A third philosopher, Schopenhauer, expresses from a different aspect the same æsthetic withdrawal from the practical urgency of life. In beauty, he says, pure knowledge reigns without effort and the beautiful does not excite the will. The beautiful thing is observed objectively and apart from all relations as the expression of an idea [269]. If the beautiful thing is ringed off, it is detached from the practical realm, as a city is isolated by its wall from ordinary attack. If " any work of fine art, anything we call beautiful, has a certain independence and completeness in itself " [270], it is withdrawn from the struggle for achievement. Mr Roger Fry repeats the same thought differently by insisting on the unity necessary for the *restful contemplation* of works of art [271], and Professor Carveth Read by emphasizing the acquisition of æsthetic value by rites and incantations that are not intended to incite to immediate action [272]. If " æsthetic appreciation ", as rendered by Mr Charles Marriott, " is dependent on the sense, which may not be conscious, of practical problems effectively *solved* " [273], it is still restfully withdrawn from practical urgency. Art, according to Miss Jane Harrison, springs " from perception and emotion that have somehow not found immediate outlet in practical action " [274].

Through differences in estimate and through differences of approach upon the æsthetic there runs a common perception of the spectatorial quality in æsthetic appreciation. As in the three hours' traffic of the stage we appreciatively observe life without sharing it, so æsthetic experience is a contemplative respite from action that has its own peculiar exhilaration. The function, or a function, of æsthetic or artistic experience is to exhilarate a partial break with active life.

Amusement, comic perception, the sense of the ludicrous, since laughter is a *complete* momentary break into relief, might seem to be the acme of æsthetic experience. Æsthetic contemplation lodged in a *partial* break, in a survey of life that is detached from practical participation without absolute loss of touch, might appear as the less developed, and the ecstasy of amused laughter that throws the laugher clean back upon himself, as the more developed, æsthetic experience. Mr Bullough, who is reluctant to admit laughter and even comedy to æsthetic status, decides that " both to laugh and to weep are direct expressions of a thoroughly practical nature, indicating almost always a concrete personal affection ". He felicitously describes the detachment of æsthetic contemplation from active life as " psychical distance ". By " psychical distance " the æsthetic object is put " out of gear with practical needs and ends " and involved in a peculiar personal relation filtered from its practical, concrete appeal, as an artist, voyaging through fog, may lose his sense of danger, cease to shrink from his clammy wrappings, and find an æsthetic joy in the colour and obscurities of his surroundings [275]. The practical appeal of the fog to the danger-instincts and feelings of discomfort is diverted into an appeal to the more contemplative æsthetic sensibilities. The fog is, as it were, held at arm's length from life, and seen, because no perception of danger numbs the seeing, to be beautiful.

But laughter seems to drop while the sense of the beautiful still holds, though at arm's length, for laughter is originally a sudden snapping of a practical tie and preserves this fundamental character in all its forms. If " the comic ", which is said to be " not co-extensive with the laughable as a whole ", apparently to admit " humour " to æsthetic status, is to be denied æsthetic rank, the denial should apparently be made because laughter breaks too violently with practical demand. Comic perception should lapse, if it does lapse, from æsthetic standing because, in Bullough's terminology, it " over-distances ", though he accuses it of " under-distancing ". Comedy, he says, is hedonic, not æsthetic : its relish derives from its " practical personal appeal " of ordinary life. Humour, for Bullough, is " distanced ridicule " : ridicule æsthetically converted from a weapon to an object of æsthetic contemplation. He should have been warned by the laugh to be wary of stretching humour on his Bed of Procrustes, for the table set on a roar is not the more quiet rapture of beauty : he has succumbed to tradition and found a permanent element of ungraciousness in the heritage of laughing. Even humour, he thinks, has fangs that have a pleasing snap though they do not bite. But when we laugh at childish naïveté, contrasting immature experience with maturity to come, there need be no ridicule, and is none if the laugher loves the child. Relief opens laughter to sympathy on the one hand even if it does open it to contempt on the other. Childish errors are amusing and need not be ridiculous, since a natural immaturity invites no logical condemnation. Childish naïveté is a great occasion for the sympathetic sense of the ludicrous most appropriately assigned to humour, and may have been one of its principal promoters.

The salvage of " humour " from the æsthetic wreck of comedy by " distancing " ridicule denotes an unsuccessful attempt to settle the æsthetic claims of laughter. If æsthetic significance proceeds from " psychical distance " it is, in one aspect, a recompense, perhaps with interest, for removal from the fervent stir of life. " Distancing " life's tyrannies sometimes extracts from them an æsthetic recompense, as Omar's

"The Flower that once has blown for ever dies"

takes its æsthetic recompense from the evanescence of life.

If "the feeling of comedy arises so far as anything which is significant or impressive, or which seems so to us, comes short, for us, of its significance or impressiveness "[276], if "the occasion of laughter is some seeming, some keeping of the word to the ear and eye, whilst it is broken to the soul "[277], comic perception may simultaneously express the break of expectancy upon incongruity and recompense for the break. The "possible comic elements" in "all embodiments of thought, passion, and volition which fall considerably below the normal standard" may be the potential recompense of expectancy which, as it rises high, is compelled to fall low. We expect great passion from a lover, even from Slender, and no mere "painful obligation of making love". So, when Slender's "love of sweet Anne Page is so faint a velleity that he is compelled to borrow all the suggestions of his passion from his uncle "[278], he bestows upon us a comic compensation for a hero of love. Little Slender, in his role of lover, masquerades as someone great. The exposure of pettiness under the imposing front of seeming grandeur is, for Lipps, the occasion of the comic [279]. If laughter is always purposeful, as though it ever sought to elate with the squanderings of gathered energies, comic perception may be the recompense for hopes foiled when rich promise ends in lean performance. If amusement is a recompense secured by laughter from broken expectations and hopes, artistic comedy may triumphantly enjoy a broken beauty. Hegel does sum up comedy as a triumph over contradictions and ruined purposes [280]. Mr Carritt, accepting from Croce the notion that æsthetic defect is a defect in expressiveness, and combining it with Hegel's hint, seeks the source of the ludicrous in the expression of an æsthetic failure in expressiveness. He is as convinced that amusement is an æsthetic satisfaction as Bullough is convinced that normally it is not, and discovers the typically amusing thing in a work of art that misses the mark. In combining triumph over hostility and incongruity into the ludicrous, he specially commends Hegel for observing that comedy is the breakdown of art, and Bergson for coming very near the truth by regarding the funny as something unsuccessfully claiming to be alive. The inclusion of triumph over hostility is apparently a deference to Plato and Hobbes, who included it in their estimates of laughter [281]. A livelier sense of the protean nature of laughter and a keener sense of the commingling of feelings in it might have prevented this marriage of triumph to pure comic sensibility. Triumph is elated and the sense of the ludicrous is elated, but two elations are not necessarily united into one. If any restriction is placed on the æsthetic status of the comic, and to admit every flash of amusement to æsthetic rank seems to be libertine liberality, the purely comic, the unpolluted sense of the ludicrous, should surely alone be included. If humour is a form of expression twice removed from the crude emotional material of life [282], being an expression of a failure to express, the inclusion of triumph in the æsthetic satisfaction of amusement at the least arouses misgivings. A clear recognition of the sympathy in humour, for Carritt seems to use "humour" as an equal equivalent for the sense of the ludicrous, for "comic", might have doubled these misgivings and perhaps have surrendered to them. Both the sympathy of humour and the triumphing of a victorious comedy may seem too participatory in life to be artistic in the narrow sense. Bullough's "distanced ridicule", which contemplates triumph without feeling it, seems nearer to the truth of humour than Carritt's triumphant sense of incongruity to the truth of comedy.

Laughter's æsthetic status is perplexing, as its instinctive status is perplexing. Its protean nature, connected with its peculiar dependence on relief, inclines it impartially towards many different classifications. It can fill with animus ; it can fill with sympathy ; it can be impartially free from both. It can arrest instincts, and simultaneously claim to be an instinctive method of interrupting them. It can make life wholesome and keep it sane ; it can also degenerate into " fun in Bagdad " and make life a chaos. Its role is most clear as an elater of situations of relief. It works ill or well according to its background : a rich life laughs richly and a petty life laughs meanly. Laughter acts and works *as if* the function had been assigned to it of making the utmost of situations of relief. The sense of the ludicrous, the characteristic and peculiar emotional accompaniment of laughter though not its only one, is intelligible in the light of this function without being fully explained.

CHAPTER XII

LAUGHTER AND REPRESSION

WHY, asks Mr Max Beerbohm, does the public
laugh when an actor has to say " damn " ?
An adequate theory of laughter, just as it
must explain why nursery tickling is laughable, must explain why this " damn " is funny
and the ludicrous element, also queried by
Mr Beerbohm, in the stage kiss and the stage
meal [283].
" If you prick us, do we not bleed ? If you
tickle us, do we not laugh ? If you poison us,
do we not die ? ; and if you wrong us, shall
we not revenge ? " The tickle and the laugh
are not as inevitably conjoined as poison and
death, though Shylock implied that they are.
His mistake is less likely to be repeated in
Max Beerbohm's three problems, for the
expletive, the kiss, and the meal are not in
themselves amusing experiences, though they
can stir the spectator to laughter. As the
laughterless tickle may become an occasion
of laughter, so damning, kissing, and eating
may provoke merriment.

LAUGHTER AND REPRESSION

A swerve of mental centering from the pseudo-reality of the stage to the reality of life is probably responsible for laughter at stage-kissing and stage-eating. The accepted illusion of the play is momentarily dropped for a suggestion of reality. Thus the kiss becomes no kiss, for the audience simultaneously expects the passion it should express and feels its make-believe. A mechanical performance masquerades as romance ; then, as attention drops from its momentary drawing towards reality into realization of counterfeit, the mask falls and amusement is stirred by the incongruity in a situation of relief. So, also, the meal becomes no meal and the audience laughs at an excessive gusto that tempts sympathetic participation high and drops it low.

The sense of the ludicrous is always ready at a play for the slipping of its leash by this swerve in mental centering. If any auditor at any moment elects to consider the incidents as though they happened in a room without losing his sense of their occurrence on a stage, he makes them ludicrous. Much ado about nothing is always potentially ludicrous if there is no serious issue, and stage traffic known to be such and judged as real life becomes simply histrionic fuss. This ludicrous contrast between apparent and simulated significance occurs more spontaneously when the dramatic quality of the play cannot continuously persuade the audience to accept the stage-illusion. A melodramatic touch is often too much for gravity : the impetuous, over-violent villain reminds expectation too forcibly that the brandished dagger is a stage gesture and that the murderous threats are repeated nightly. In some moods the stage pageant is fiercely contrasted with the urgency of life :

> "What's Hecuba to him or he to Hecuba
> That he should weep for her ? "

Hamlet was too impassioned to be amused ; in happier moods the importunity of wild stage-tears is ludicrous if it stirs a contrast between what should be grief and is not.

The stage-oath is probably accepted precisely as it would be accepted off the stage and comic for the same reason as an oath in ordinary life is comic. Relief by mental explosion is the essence of the " damn ". Laughter is thus provided with its fundamental situation. The spectator receives the principal benefit from this fundamental situation, since his secondhand feeling of relief is more free from the annoyance that may curb laughter in the swearer. His sense of incongruity is also heightened as if the commination service had been read over a teasing fly. The theological anathema of the oath is preserved in the sentiment against its use, though the explicit meaning is lost in its simple use as an expletive, and the sense of relief is also heightened by a sense of escape from conventional repression. If outraged sentiment does not forbid laughter, the flouting of a public ban incites in the spectator a joyous sense of freedom from repression, and the oath is hailed as an escape from bondage. If the stage-oath is more freely comic than a real oath it is because it provokes less easily public resentment against it. The actor is permitted to swear as he is permitted to murder—because he does not really do it. The relieved discharge of the oath and its incongruous occurrence in despite of public ban is an example of the ludicrous in relief from repression. There seems to be abundance of relief in the oath : it scatters a gathered anger, defies a public convention, and may also suggest to the spectator an attack which fails to mature by converting a blow into an expletive.

The " damn " theory of laughter, if picturesque rather than accurate definition is allowed for the moment, is now enjoying a vogue. So far as a " damn " is letting out something that should be, or is actually being, kept in, it is typical of the " letting the cat out of the bag " by which Holt describes Freud's theory of wit and humour [284].

Witticisms, according to Freud, are successful escapes from suppression. Harmless wit revels in absurdities and plausible nonsense that soothe the protest of reason : thoughts are wittily disguised to deceive judgment and escape from its critical ban, as they masquerade in dreams to slip past the " censor ". " Tendency-wit " indulges either an attack that without its witty expression would remain a suppressed hostility or a verbal exposure of the indecent that would otherwise remain an ungratified wish. Wit eludes a hindrance and secures pleasure from sources that would be inaccessible, through repression, without its aid. Witty expression makes childish playful nonsense worthy of an adult, for he can talk like a child if he can wittily persuade reason that he speaks like a man. The hostile man can satisfy his animus if he disarms his enemy and gratifies his audience by the wittiness of his attack. The man who is partial to indecency can talk freely of it if he speaks wittily. Thus the lover of juvenile irresponsibility or of belligerency or of the obscene can indulge his preference if he can summon enough wit to break through the restriction imposed upon him by good sense or good manners. He can be silly or impolite or rebellious or bitter or indecent if he can be witty enough to parry the censure he would incur if he were any of these without being witty as well.

" Tendency-wit ", serving hostility or indecency, develops out of an original and juvenile wit of playful childish irresponsibility.

This original wit secures its pleasure from its technique, which is essentially economical. It is economical by condensing joyous festivities into " alcoholidays " or by double meaning in Douglas Jerrold's ascription to a father who had cut off his heir with a shilling of *" unremitting* kindness " or by other carefully specified methods. When Freud remarks that wit saves nothing by its technique because it laboriously searches for its words and imitates the housewife who spends time and money on transit to buy vegetables where they are a cent cheaper, he does not seem to realize fully that its essence is decisiveness, usually secured in part by conciseness, of expression. The final sword-stroke is decisive, and results in victory though the duel and the victor's apprenticeship to swordsmanship may have been long. Though he seems for the most part to recognize the importance of brevity for the witticism, he does not sufficiently recognize the higher functions of wit. " Tendency-wit " derives pleasure, like playful wit, from its technique and adds to it the satisfaction of a gratified and repressed tendency [285]. The witty illumination of a truth, which need not fear scrutiny from reason nor be a pretext for either hostility or indecency, is very incompletely recognized. " Experience is a good schoolmaster, but the school-fees are somewhat heavy " is both good wit and good sense : it has a poignant sense of truth, contains no hostile stab, and has no relish of the indecent.

Freud's theory of wit centres, and, it may be added, centres too exclusively, on the providing of laughter with its situation of relief by the release of a repression. The joy of wit and the emotion suffusing its laughter, so far as it does laugh, should depend on the gratification of suppressed tendencies—wit results in something resembling triumph and the enjoyment of it. Mr Eastman accuses Freud of an awkward attempt to combine this estimate with a theory of economized psychic energy and of contriving an ill-assorted alliance between himself, Herbert Spencer, and Lipps—discharge of surplus energy being the formula for laughter adopted by his two injudiciously selected allies [286]. Greig remarks, less disapprovingly, that Freud's theory of wit is not, and should not be considered as, a complete theory of laughter. " For Freud ", he adds, " wit is one thing, the comic another, and humour a third " [287]. Eastman's criticism perhaps touches a muddling in Freud's application of one formula to the witty, the comic, and the humorous : " The pleasure of wit originates from an economy of expenditure in inhibition, of the comic from an economy of an expenditure in thought, and of humour from an economy of an expenditure in feeling " [288]. Economized inhibition seems to be a muddled description of a witticism that releases hostility from repression by the force of its wit. Economized energy also seems a curious description of the comic in a clown who fusses round a circus without doing anything. Laughter is a spill-way for the dissipation of expectant preparation, as when, to use one of Freud's own illustrations, a clown plants himself firmly to catch a very light ball. If " economized " energy means energy applied to securing comic or humorous effect when it is not required for its original purpose, wit has been forcibly fitted into the common formula. Freud himself contrasts wit with comic effect as " made " to " found ". Without arguing the point, without attempting to follow the intricacies of Freud's thought, or without suggesting that wit economizes expenditure by substituting satirical attack for a blow, it should be noted that for Freud wit *is* different from comic laughter. He seems to be aware, though his sense of the fact may be disturbed and even vague, that wit, through its decisiveness, may provide the situation of relief so fundamental and essential to laughter. In quoting Fischer's " the judgment which produces the comic contrast is wit " [289], and in referring to Lipps' connection of wit with a " conscious and clever evocation of the comic " [290], Freud hints at the provision by wit of the incongruity that gives to comic perception its opportunity. He hovers round the conception of the sense of the ludicrous as the more purely mental analogue of the more purely physical situation of relief. As the laughter of triumph arises when success calls off gathered energies and drops into sudden relief, so comic laughter arises when excited expectancy is suddenly relieved from its tension, though its perception of an incongruity, of a contrast administering a psychical shock that contains relief and a relieved pleasure, charges it with its own specific emotion of amusement. He suggests that the comic effect is a difference between two expenditures of energy, the one of " feeling one's self into something " and the other of an actual expenditure by the ego. We perceive an energetic (and futile) clown and the difference between our own sympathetic realization of his physical energy and our own private mental diminution of it by simply perceiving or thinking of it creates a contrast between too much in the physical and too little in the mental. He hardly seems to recognize the importance of the *futile* element in such comic effects : we expect great results from the clown's vigour and discover very little ones.

Humorous laughter, as understood in these chapters, permits the ready diffusion of sympathy rather than economizes it as in Freud's estimate [291]. The main significance of Freud's contribution, from the point of view maintained in this book, is the emphasis upon release of repression as one begetter of the situation of incongruous relief that generates laughter. Miss Bliss also emphasizes release of repression, though she places it in a different setting. Civilization imposes restraints on the natural man, who laughs when he suddenly escapes from them [292]. Belligerent wit as construed by Freud and laughter as " a return to nature " as Miss Bliss construes it, have a certain resemblance to an imprecatory " damn ". Without pressing the comparison of these released repression theories to the expletive or dwelling on their relation to the " unconscious " or the " subconscious ", which is an important item in modern " repression " doctrines, they may be observed to circle round the fundamental conception of relief that provides an adequate mental standpoint for regarding laughter. Release of repression is obviously one method of securing relief and stimulating amused laughing by an incongruity. It is also a particular instance of the method of laughter. Laughter pleasantly breaks off an activity ; it relaxes an unrequired effort, whether more exclusively in the physical sphere as in sheer laughter of relief or more exclusively in the mental sphere as in comic laughter ; when it breaks the pressure of inhibition it pleasantly interrupts the " effort " of repression. Laughter arises when gathered energies are suddenly called off, and the relief of released repression adds one more illustration of the " many waters " in which the " oare " of laughter dips.

A sympathetic sense of escape from repression laughs when Mr Charles Chaplin, observing a fine lady haughtily staring at him through her lorgnette, steps up to her and slaps her face. Convention forbids him to slap — but he does it. The comic sense, always adding its own gusto to the laughable situation, revels also in the incongruity of an expected deference in the actor, expected because social convention ordains it, and an actual rudeness. Charlie says " damn you " with his hand. He should not do it, but, when he does, the act is ludicrous. A satisfaction over a ruffling of dignified rudeness also helps the ludicrous situation along. Mr Charles Chaplin, according to Mr Eastman, ascribes his comic effects to " telling them the plain truth about things " : the fine lady deserves a slap, and she gets it. Now we may be, as Eastman says, " always hungry for the simple truth " [293], but we are not necessarily amused when we get it, any more than we necessarily laugh when we eat. The truth-telling theory of laughter, or comic laughter, is only partial, for only some truths and only some methods of telling them are funny. A student will probably laugh or smile if told that he has passed his examination, but, though he hears the "simple truth", he will not laugh, or only smile the rueful smile that is no smile, if told that he has not passed. Truth and truth-telling are not inherently laughable or comic. An unexpected home-truth may be funny if it disconcerts the victim, not because truth is funny but because he gets something he did not expect. Mr Chaplin's slap is funny because the slappee suddenly and forcibly realizes how very annoyed he is. It is funny because the audience sympathetically realizes the relief, so predisposing to laughter, of a vented annoyance, and, expecting conventional if strained politeness, observes an unconventional slap.

The laughter of the situation of relief through relieved repression, like laughter arising out of other reliefs, may suffuse its sense of the ludicrous with other feelings. A critic of the leisured classes might satisfy his animus in the Chaplin slap and satisfy it more if it occurred in real life. So also repressed contempt or repressed scorn or repressed self-importance may empty themselves in a laugh.

Wit can provide laughter with its situation, and repression, when sharply relieved, is one distinct, and perhaps important, contributor to those breaks into relief from which the laugh arises.

CHAPTER XIII

SUMMARY AND CONCLUSION

LAUGHTER makes no secret of its infinite variety. Almost any joke can be taken in many different ways and relished in many different spirits.

> *Lady :* " So you don't believe in politics, Giles ? "
> *Gardener :* " Yes, mum, I does, just as I believe in the wire-worm—you can't 'elp it when you sees the mischief they do." [294]

This joke may be taken ludicrously, as a sheer amused delight in the double turn given to the inquirer's expectation—first onto an emphatic, unanticipated belief and secondly on to a disconcerting reason for it. A confirmed politician or political enthusiast might relish its comic aspect without even a slight sense of sting. An anti-political orator might insist on the sting ; in the heat of controversy the joke might be resented as a blow and answered with one. Laughter at this joke may be purely comic, or amusedly and playfully enjoy a " dig ", or it may be openly derisive.

SUMMARY AND CONCLUSION

A jest's prosperity lies in the ear that hears it ; its character also depends on the spirit that takes it. Laughter can be unfairly suspected of derision or of cruelty when it is merely exuberant or appreciative of the comic because the occasion, as in stage quips or buffetings, *could* gratify a cruel or derisive laugh. Derision-theories of laughter have perhaps sometimes failed to perceive that what could be derision or cruelty is, in the laughable occasion, in actual fact comic. The possibility of suspecting ungracious elements in jokes relished for their ludicrous zest and the possibility of enjoying them cruelly or triumphantly or contemptuously indicate that laughter can be scornful or triumphant or cruel.

It seems clear that laughter can wholeheartedly express battle-triumph or be filled with scorn or self-congratulation. It seems equally clear that the purely genial laughter of greeting or the hilarious laughter of play is different from the ungracious laughters on the one hand and from comic laughter on the other. Sheer relief also seems to be a species of laughter. Though these feelings or emotions mingle, their mingling can be realized and their separate natures distinguished. Since sympathy seems obvious in some laughs and anti-sympathetic feelings in others, the act of laughing seems to be a *rendez-vous* for very various emotions. The laughter of greeting alone is a troublesome occurrence for theories of laughter that are too exclusive in their definitions. Laughter seems to insist on its own variety and to demand a " formula or set of formulæ " for some " things in general " such as Mr Max Beerbohm deprecates [295]. His deprecation is intelligible if the while richness of laughter is expected in the formula. A single formula can never wholly contain many things or one of them. But the collection of many laughters round the single act of laughing or smiling and their free mingling round that " mechanical motion " suggests a fundamental situation common to all laughs from which they all spring.

Laughter also seems to be a very sensitive thing. The ways men laugh and the things they laugh at are excellent indexes of their natures. Anger is resistant to sympathy. It may be controlled by its *milieu*—indulged, for example, where morals are undisciplined, and restricted where they are not ; but it is not in itself sympathetic. Laughter freely admits sympathy or animus. The sensitiveness of laughter to the character, circumstances, and experience of the laugher and the many varieties it displays can be connected with one fundamental element that systematizes the laughters into a single well defined group.

The richness of variety in laughter has tempted many to exclaim against attempts to refer its varieties to a single source and the rich variety of theories tempts to belief in their protests. But there must be some fundamental connection between all experiences that announce themselves " physically in the pleasant spasms we call laughter ". There must be some mental standpoint which secures the varieties of laughter, its numerous occasions and all interpretations of its nature that have any degree of discernment in a single perspective. This standpoint is attained and the perspective secured by observing the fundamental plan of which all laughters are variants. The mechanics of laughter hints very plainly at this fundamental plan. This hint has been accepted restrictively and laughter confined to one emotion. But M°Dougall's restriction of laughter to the one specific emotion of amusement does not mislead a clear realization of the emotional variety in laughter, and the distinct hint in the mechanics of laughter then reveals a common character in the many laughters.

The " happy convulsion " of laughter occurs in a situation of relief. It collapses the laugher into a stationary exerciser of his own body who is convulsively withdrawn from intervention in the active affairs of life. It marks the sudden relaxation of unrequired effort, and its repetitive series of respiratory explosions or tremulation of body, more vigorously or more quietly, rehearses an original situation in which a call upon effort is sharply called off. The original, more physical situation of the laugher is too plainly exposed in the motions of his body to be mistaken. As a spring firmly pressed against an obstacle vibrates when the obstacle is withdrawn, so the body shakes to and fro, with gasps in its breathing, in tremulous laughter, when its effort suddenly relaxes into relief. A quick interruption of activity that precipitates into relief is the essential characteristic of laughter as it is revealed in its characteristic bodily expression. Laughter is a *diversion*—a pleasant expenditure upon the body of energy released from other activities.

The physical act of laughing clearly invites an ample interpretation of the nature of laughter and warns the theorist against confining it too narrowly. "The laugh thus marks an interruption to the behaviour of love which has been overcome with a less expenditure of energy than was originally prepared for the purpose "[296]. It may mark the interruption of *any* behaviour and is not confined to "overcoming". The exultant laugh of triumph or elated laughter over sudden success rejoices in overcoming but the sudden *withdrawal* of a menace results in a laugh that has no sense of victory. The sense of the ludicrous that steadily tends to suffuse all laughter with amusement has perhaps a freer scope in laughters which have little sense of conquest. Overcoming is apt to fill the laugh with triumph or with some more genial gusto of gratified accomplishment. The interval of relief, in which laughter arises, is closely connected with play and is apt to arise sharply and repeatedly in the hilarious or holiday mood. Since laughter is always a momentary holiday, a relaxation, it is appropriate to the mental mood that reaches its height in the spirit of carnival. Many thinkers have hovered round this connection between laughter and play—often perilously, for they have succumbed to the temptation of construing laughter too narrowly by confining it to a connection with play. The interval of relief, in which laughter arises, is also closely connected with seriousness. The highest laughter, indeed, is a momentary lapse from earnestness. Since play itself is often serious and may, as when men begin playing golf in the intervals of business and end by doing business in the intervals of golf, become more serious than more important activities, it is not the indispensable genial source of all laughters. Play may make itself comic by an overplus of seriousness, as golf and other sports would often make the gods on Olympus laugh, if they were there to laugh, by the enthusiasm and diligence to which they frequently stir their devotees. But neither play nor more important endeavour is the sole or essential *milieu* of laughter.

Laughter is an interjection into the behaviour of human beings and is apt to be interjected whenever relaxation occurs through the interruption of unrequired effort. It may be genially interjected into ungenial behaviour. Two boys faced one another with angry looks : a fight was rapidly accumulating in their words and gestures. Suddenly a small onlooker perceived the ludicrous in the situation and laughed. The laugh spread through the group of onlooking boys and then, probably unintentionally on their part and perhaps to their chagrin, for boys delight in a fight, promptly incapacitated the two opponents from fighting by spreading to them. This little incident is an effective warning against the assumption that, because play and laughter are both genial moods, they have an inseparable or even a specially close connection. Play occurs in the intervals between more serious matters and in this sense is relaxation. But since laughter, as is written on its physical manifestation, is an absolute relaxation, a dropping into relief, a break in action, there is no more necessary a connection between laughter and play than there is between laughter and any form of activity. Play and the carnival mood usually permit situations of relief to occur freely : to this extent laughter and holidays may be said to have a special connection. Business is constantly calling for effort and sustaining the call ; holidays free the laugher from such a sustained call on his energies and allow him to drop frequently into the relief situation of laughter. But laughter may be interjected whenever and wherever a call upon effort is suddenly called off into relief.

The relaxation of the laugh is an invitation to all appropriate emotions : to triumph when relief comes from a sword-thrust or other stroke of achievement, to scorn when the call of a threat is sharply followed by a sense of its futility, to greeting when the tension of social intercourse drops at the discovery of a friend. The most original emotional accompaniment of the laugh is probably sheer relief, and is associated with the most physical form of the occasion of laughter. Its relieved relaxation both opens it to sympathy and allows animus to linger. Thus laughter is always protean—impartially hospitable to many emotions and maintaining the integrity of society by the double method of linking its members in sympathy and correcting their faults by ridicule, or the fear of it. It can be bitter or sweet, even both in a breath : it can embrace or discard, and be gracious or ungracious. It is pleasant in itself, since it is the sign of relief or respite, though it may derisively plant a dagger in a breast

as well as share a joy. Its protean nature
has been a source of misconceptions, for as
Proteus of old might be mistaken now for a
timid deer and now for a raging boar, according to his momentary shape, so laughter has
been misunderstood by partial perceptions
of its many characters. Mr Greig rightly
insists on the " relativity of laughter " [297].
In vindictive or cruel epochs vindictiveness
or cruelty will tinge or dominate laughter.
As civilization restrains animus or secures
one man from another's violence, laughter
reflects its progress and stands more open to
sympathy. As sympathy increases, laughter
is more and more prompted by occasions in
which sympathetic linkage is possible or
remains unbroken and less and less prompted
by occasions involving misery or cruelty or
misfortune.

The adult tends to laugh differently from
the child. A row of spectators at a tennis-
match included adults and both young girls
and boys. When an elderly lady tripped over
the guy-rope that supported a net-pole and
fell there was a sharp contrast between the
giggle that ran through the young folk and
the seriousness of their elders. The difference
depended on the absence or presence of a sense
of the seriousness of a fall for an elderly lady.
Experience of life alters the occasions of
laughter and so does the sense of sympathy.
This episode clearly illustrates the dependence

of laughter upon the *milieu* for obtaining its situation of relief.

Laughter is your true catholic who mixes with all. Its catholicity has led to misunderstanding through its . association with tickling. " If you prick us, do we not bleed ? if you tickle us, do we not laugh ? if you poison us, do we not die ? and if you wrong us, shall we not revenge ? " Circumspect scrutiny avoids Shylock's error—the assertion of as inevitable a connection between laughter and tickling as between death and poison. For the act of laughing, which is not an act *by* but *within* the body, is different from the squirm of the tickle. The laugh, which collapses the laugher, cannot be the proper response to the tickle, which is always an *act of riddance*. The sneeze rids the nostrils of irritants ; the cough does the like for the throat ; and tickling ensures for both the occurrence of the appropriate act of riddance. Whether the squirm in the nursery tickle was impressed upon the male to ensure vigorous struggling in battle or upon the maiden to repel the advances of a too importunate lover or upon both to twitch off parasites, whether the tickled wriggle is a wrestle, a refusal of love [298], or a " bug-shifter " [299], it is always an act of riddance and essentially different from the absence of endeavour in the laugh. The tickle, in nursery tickling, simply offers an occasion for laughter. The act of riddance is more violent than the situation demands. The tickle stimulates as though the tickler were hostile—it calls fiercely on the body for action. Since the occasion is friendly and not hostile, the fierce call on drops into a relative call off, relative because the child still shrinks from the tickling hand though his first impulse to resent real hostility quickly wanes, and a situation of relief provides laughter with its occasion.

The sense of the ludicrous hints at its connection with laughter of sheer relief and with other laughters where the body is clearly involved by attaching itself to the same physical expression of laughing. It is the more purely mental analogue of the more purely physical situation of sheer relief. Drawing the distinction between mental and bodily more sharply than really warrants, for there is a mental element in the most purely bodily form of laughter as the body is never quite forgotten in the most purely ludicrous sense, the experience of the comic repeats in the mental sphere the experience of relief in sudden relaxations of bodily effort. A call on attention, or expectation —and attention usually contains an expectant element, called off into relief where it is momentarily freed from any other obligation than to relish the perception of the incongruity, is the occasion of the ludicrous. An incongruity is a contrast that administers a psychical shock and a ludicrous incongruity is lodged in a situation of relief. The parallel between the woman who laughed when she was plucked from the machine and the listener who laughed at the fall of the lake level when the angler pulled out his fish is clear and complete. The one was called upon for struggle, the other for understanding. In both the call was cut short and both were dropped into relief—the woman because danger was over and the angler's auditor because narration had forfeited its claim on belief. The sheer relief of the one had its analogue in the amusement of the other.

The analogy between laughter at the ludicrous and laughter from sheer relief can admit a wide difference between the two laughters. Analogous situations may be very different variants of one fundamental plan or system of connections. As an oak grows from vital factors concentrated in an acorn, so civilizations have grown from concentrations of resources in isolated peoples. The fundamental factor—isolation—has been effected by different methods. The sea has isolated and the desert has isolated. " The bordering desert ", remarks Miss Newbigin in this connection, " ensured isolation, and, continuing the island metaphor, we may say that it represented the sea. Its effect was to throw the whole energy of the community towards the centre, for the periphery formed an area in which the characteristic mode of life could not be practised. Similarly, it gave protection, for it is unsuited to any save a highly specialized culture, which must have been of relatively late origin " [300]. Two peoples, one encircled by sea and the other by sand, are in different but analogous situations. But the variations of a fundamental situation may be widely divergent. Response to environment is a fundamental relation of life. Animal forms present a bewildering multiplicity because the lower animals usually respond to their environment by changing their bodies. This " direct structural response " may have occurred in early human history " when man reacted to the sum total of the conditions as an animal does ". Man's present response, however, is communal and his " real response to the surface phenomena of the earth " is " the aptitudes which the members of a community display, the tools which they use, the kind of knowledge which they accumulate, their modes of organization, their type of material wealth, their traditions and ideals " [301]. Animals respond to their environment by changing their bodies ; men by changing their tools and their ideas. Both participate in the situation of responding to their environment, but civilization is very different from structural changes in animal bodies. So the sense of the ludicrous is very different from sheer relief, though the fundamental plan or situation is identical in both, as response to environment is the fundamental plan or situation underlying variety of animal species on the one hand and the variety of civilizations on the other.

Though the sense of the ludicrous may disguise its connection with obviously relieved laughters, like those of triumph or superiority, and prompt suspicion about its natural analogy with the laugh of sheer relief, it announces that connection and that analogy by one significant character. Every laugh is a momentary finality, and, as laughter of sheer relief ends effort, so the point of a joke is a terminus. Ridicule is rhetorically powerful because it uproariously makes further inquiry impossible : " Gorgias laid it down rightly enough as a sound maxim to confound the seriousness of one's adversary by jocularity " [302]. So with pure amusement : the book closes and the chapter ends. Sheer relief, triumph, scorn, greeting, and amusement—all these laughs are momentary termini, breaks in the flow, elated and suddenly precipitated respites.

If the call changes so that there is no terminus, the laugh is spoiled : a sudden sense of danger will quickly dissipate amusement. Comic laughter, like all laughter, essentially

announces and relishes a situation of relief :
it is a momentary terminus.

Amusement is peculiar to laughter because
it is the appreciation of an incongruity lodged
in the characteristic relief-situation of the
laugh. It rises in connection with the laugh,
tends to suffuse it, and constantly dominates
it, because the break in relief *is* an incongruity
whose perception and appreciation compose
the comic sense. Amusement creeps into the
laugh of triumph or scorn, and is immanent
from the first in all human laughter, because
the incongruous sides of every break into
relief tend to engage the perception and
appreciation of incongruity. In purely comic
laughter the situation is purely mental
(cutting mental and bodily more sharply
asunder than in reality, for the sake of
analysis) and amused laughter, sensitive like
all laughters to emotions appropriate to
relief from tension, by admitting sympathy
with its relaxation from hostility, can become
humour—the final achievement of the laugh.
Amusement can allow animus to linger ; it
can even invite it by contemptuous indifference ; but it tends to soften the asperity of
ungracious laughter by emphasizing and enlivening the relaxation of relief. Amusement
itself has no animus and tends to displace it,
though the two may co-exist and the satirist
may doubly spice his gibe with the ludicrous
and the contemptuous.

Laughter may obtain its relief from the sudden call off of a call on that is either momentary or persistent. Serious occasions claim sustained seriousness and, as dust-particles act as nuclei for the condensation of rain, trivial interruptions at a funeral often drop sustained mental tension into quick relief and indecorous laughter. In the nursery tickle the call on and the call off are both rapid. Release of tension is the thing, whether the tension has lasted an hour or a second. Prolonged tension tends to search for laughter, or for the relief that it marks, and a moment of fierce emotion, as it trembles from vigour, is ready for respite.

When Homer made the bandy-legged Thersites, lame-footed, his rounded shoulders arched over his chest and his head with its scanty sprouting stubble warped over them, a reviler who was hateful to Achilles and Odysseus [303], he commemorated a traditional ascription of bitterness to the person with deformity or physical infirmity. So Richard, " not shap'd for sportive tricks ", brought " into this breathing world, scarce half made up " and halting past the barking dogs, resolved " to prove a villain " and be " subtle, false, and treacherous " [304]. This traditional connection between deformity and bitterness was established by the unsympathetic laughter aroused by the former. Physical infirmities easily excited ancient laughter. Plato was shocked when Homer describes how

"Inextinguishable laughter arose among the blessed gods, when they saw Hephæstus bustling about the mansion" [305].

Hephæstus limped as he bustled and, nearer to our own day, Thackeray could say of Pope that " his contemporaries reviled these misfortunes with a strange acrimony and made his poor deformed person the butt for many a bolt of heavy wit " [306]. If the reviled turned reviler, who could blame him ? If the deformed were legitimate objects of mirth, who could condemn their bitterness ? The passing of the tradition that deformity is bitter marks an alteration to a sympathetic attitude towards the ill-shaped person. This change of attitude is reflected in the history of the laugh, for deformity is no longer a legitimate occasion of mirth. Here sympathy has checked the laugh : the expectancy of normal humanity is broken by the spectacle of infirmity, and laughter follows if derisive or contemptuous feelings permit relief ; but the call to expect normality is more altered to a call for sympathy in the modern civilized mind than called off into the relief of laughter that may blend scorn with amusement. A relic of the flow of the comic sense at the sight of deformity is preserved in Bergson's comment that a hunchback is comic because he suggests a man cultivating a rigid attitude, and in his comparison of the comic expression to " a unique and permanent grimace " [307]. It is, perhaps, suggestive that Aristotle, in his most frequently quoted passage on the ridiculous, chooses the mask as an instance of excitants of laughter [308] : the mask clearly hints at the absurdity and also, perhaps, at the opportunity for derision, naturally suggested by physical infirmity. Traill [309] places the human tendency to laugh at deformity side by side with its suppression by sympathy when he reminds us of the part played in the fun of the fair by grinning through a horse-collar, and that Persius, the Roman satirist, condemned the man who could taunt another on the loss of an eye.

Sympathy has restricted laughter by depriving it of an occasion in deformity, and Groos affirms that both danger and sympathy prevent the enlivening effect of the comic [310]. Another writer [311] defines humour as " a more subtle, delicately discriminating sense of incongruity " and dubs the " sympathetic feature in humour " as " somewhat accidental " : humour is the sense of the ludicrous at its height—super-amusement, and " too much emphasis " must not be laid upon its sympathy. The restrictions imposed upon laughter by sympathy account for these opinions, but do not justify their lack of insight. For sympathies permit laughter as well as refuse it. Aristotle knew we can be

fond of persons " who have a certain amount
of tact in giving and receiving badinage, as,
whether they are good-humoured butts or
graceful jesters, they have the same object
in view as the opposite parties in the combat
of wit, viz. mutual amusement " [312]. The
sympathies between members of a friendly
circle can allow a jest or a witticism that
would be cruel and ostracized for its cruelty
if mutual good-feeling and fellowship did not
" distance " the ridicule. Thus sympathy
sometimes permits laughter as well as denies
it, and it can suffuse the rich, genial laugh of
humour.

Groos thinks that a feeling of superiority
livens up the comic, in contradistinction to
sympathy which chills its liveliness. Mr
Carritt apparently combines the ludicrous of
triumph and incongruity : " Hence the element of triumph over something hostile, noted
in it by Plato and Hobbes, and the element
of incongruity and incoherence noted
by others " [313]. Superiority and triumph, in
all its varieties — noble or ignoble, battle-
triumph or intellectual satisfaction over
mental achievement—are not hinderers of
the laugh. They are too appropriate to its
fundamental situation of relief to restrict it
as sympathy restricts it, and they have
undoubtedly always haunted it. Their haunting habit has been restricted by sympathy
and also, as previously suggested, by the sheer

excluding force of the sense of the ludicrous which has more and more tended to enliven the laugh and to wean laughter from its dependence for gusto on the gratification either of success or of animus. A sense of the appropriateness of superiority or triumph to the general situation of laughter has been partly responsible for a clinging by theorists to ungracious estimates of the nature of laughter. The frequent animus in the laugh has tightened their hold on this estimate. The possibility of construing purely comic jokes—jokes made and taken in only a ludicrous spirit—into indulgence of animus has prevented this tightened hold from relaxing. The theorists who appeal to Hobbes or for whom he is spokesman have perceived the truth partially. Gratified animus is emotionally congruent with the relief of the laughable situation—so congruent that it persistently haunts it. The humanization of laughter, perceptible in its history, intimates plainly that gratified animus is not essential to its occurrence. If superiority is contrasted with gratified animus as self-satisfaction with hostile attention to a fellow, neither is it essential. Laughter has many varieties—perhaps even including the laugh of " mental vacuity " [314]. Accepting for expository convenience the clean Cartesian cut between mind and body, " the laugh of the soul and the laugh of the body are distinct.

We may have each without the other. And only a gross and superficial analysis will confound them " [315]. Many different feelings may *rendez-vous* about the laugh. They are often ungracious, and purely comic laughter may be dispassionately free from either animus or sympathy, but Pater rightly identified humour, certainly the highest humour, with " the laughter which blends with tears, and even with the subtleties of the imagination, and which, in its most exquisite motives, is one with pity. . . ." [316]. Dan Leno graphically described an explosion in his home. " It was the only time ", he added, " that father and mother went out together ". This joke has no cutting edge, and has been rightly described as humorous in its sympathetic presentation of the ludicrous, though an unsympathetic critic of marital relations might relish it as a gibe.

Laughter has steadily replaced triumph by amusement, though it has not banished it, and it has opened to sympathy, though it has not completely expelled animus. It has also genialized triumph and attracted gratification at success that has discarded hostility. The quiet laugh that greets the decisiveness of wit is the laugh of triumph without its animus. It has not necessarily developed out of the latter, for many laughters may spring from the central situation of relief, as many rays of light diverge from a luminous point.

SUMMARY AND CONCLUSION

The sedater form of pleasurable emotion assigned by Traill [317] to wit as its natural response and evoked by a double sense of fitness and human ingenuity is, so far as it employs the laugh, a laughter of achievement that may correspond to the laugh of battle-triumph without being its lineal descendant. The two laughters may be analogues : the triumphant laugh having the same relation to a decisive sword-stroke as the " sedate emotion " has to witty and decisive exposure of truth. Nor need the sense of humour have had, as Traill affirms—following a tradition—an anti-pathetic origin [318]. If the sense of the ludicrous, as Traill's sense of " humour " must be rechristened under present terminology, originated in a perception of incongruity and was nourished by relishing it, it sprang, like triumph, from a situation of relief but had its own private route of development. The laughters are more like children of relief, each separately born, than like a straight step-by-step series in which each member is a modification of the one before it.

As the laugh varies with its originating relief so it may vary with the purpose of the witticism. The triumphant laugh of aggressive or satirical wit has an echo of war, and scorn or contempt or superiority may tinge laughter according to the relief precipitated. The laughter of wit sometimes quietly appreciates an achievement of insight and expression ;

sometimes it has the relish of the stirred sense of the ludicrous. The quality of the relief promotes a corresponding quality in the laugh and the witticism, because it varies the situation of relief, varies the gusto of laughter. Wit attracts the phrase " laughter of wit " because it so often and so competently provides the laughters with occasions. Its decisiveness elicits their fundamental situation of relief and it constantly involves those displays of incongruity that stir the sense of the ludicrous. The alliance between wit and laughter, frequent though not constant, is a reminder of the ubiquity of the laugh. It is ubiquitous because sudden interruptions of unrequired effort constantly recur. They recur because quirks and stoppages are ever interjecting into the flow of human life. The sense of the ludicrous is invasive of the laugh because incongruities stir it, and pervasive simply because this is a changing universe. For " incongruity ", as Mr Santayana remarks, " is a consequence of change ", and " existence involves changes and happenings and is comic inherently, like a pun that begins with one meaning and ends with another " [319].

" In youth ", adds Mr Santayana, " anything is pleasant to see or do, so long as it is spontaneous, and if the conjunction of these things is ridiculous, so much the better : to be ridiculous is part of the fun ". Such addition to hilarity, in which amusement adds to the fun, bespeaks the function of the comic. Laughter is the elater of relief and, as the more patently physical laughters enliven respites from physical action, so the ludicrous sense enlivens respites from comprehension. There has been diligent search for the function of the laugh. It has been too narrowed simultaneously into an expression exclusively of amusement and a saviour from unnecessary sympathy. It has been too undiscriminatingly assigned a " strong survival value " : there are other incentives than the extraction of laughing satisfaction to quick perceptions of significant distinctions, and it is doubtful whether the *incongruities* that excite laughter ever assisted a human being directly in the battle of life [320]. Laughter may have more indirectly contributed to survival by its periodical enlivenments of heart and soul. For this enlivenment seems to be its essential and primary function and it is too intimately blended with the sense of the ludicrous for this essential and primary function to require further search. There may be a spread of function from this primary role of enlivenment, as the qualities of laughter spread from its primary quality of relief. The laughing relish of absurdities in conduct reacts in the social discipline of ridicule upon the perpetrators of the absurdities. The elation of kindly laughter spreads as a sympathetic bond. Laughter varies its function as it varies its nature and it can divide by bitterness as it can join by sympathy. It does all these things—dealing out discipline, sowing discord, and genially uniting. But its central, fundamental role, from which other effects secondarily spring, is the enlivenment of those breaks or momentary termini that constantly recur in human activity and supply laughter with its generative respite.

Though the æsthetic status of laughter, comic laughter, is as difficult to define as its position among the instincts, it can take its recompense of amusement from the contradictions and bafflements of life as the poet or artist can take his contemplative recompense from the urgency of existence. "What shadows we are, and what shadows we pursue"!—thus the dying Walpole, by expressing his sense of the vanity of life, took his æsthetic recompense from evanescence. So Burns took his in:—

"But pleasures are like poppies spread,
  You seize the flower, its bloom is shed;
  Or, like the snow-fall in the river,
  A moment white, then melts for ever."

The comic spirit may suffuse cynicism or bitterness with the enlivenment of amusement, or, on the level of humour, it may laugh

224

over the contradictions of life with a quickened sense of sympathy. The course of true love is not the only course of life that does not run smoothly, and humorous laughter can extract a recompense from frequent breaks between human actualities and ideals without either quenching humanity or unnerving endeavour. . . . " Hence the best of all jokes is the sympathetic contemplation of things by the understanding from the philosopher's point of view. There is no joke so true and deep in actual life as when some pure idealist goes up and down among the institutions of society, attended by a man who knows the world, and who, sympathizing with the philosopher's scrutiny, sympathizes also with the confusion and indignation of the detected skulking institutions. His perception of disparity, his eye wandering perpetually from the rule to the crooked, lying, thieving fact, makes the eyes run over with laughter " [321].

But life is not all comedy and, though " men of reason " may have been unreasonably denied the spirit of joking by Emerson [321], they do not permanently regard it as comedy. Fuller included " jesting " in the " Holy State " but only when it was not " a master-quality " and " attended on other perfections " [322]. The continuous insistence on life as a comic pageant tends to a combination of Olympian aloofness with quiet contempt.

SUMMARY AND CONCLUSION

Aristotle approved "the perfect mean of virtue" between the buffoon who "is the slave of his own merriment" and "cannot refrain from deriding either himself or others" and the morose, sour person who does not joke and is irritated with those who do. "Perfect humour", he adds, should include both cleverness and tact, and thus befit "a considerate and right-minded gentleman". The lighter innuendo of the New Comedy was more decorous, he continues, than the scurrility and obscenity of the Old. He thus notes a humanization of the laugh and urges its refinement. But he significantly remarks that "the joke is of the nature of a taunt" [323]. When, as his description of comedy as "an imitation of men worse than the average" with respect to one particular fault, the ridiculous [324], may be roughly taken to indicate, he contrasted the upward look in tragedy with the downward look in comedy, he originated a very persistent tradition.

"Do you know", writes Oliver Wendell Holmes—mildly retaining an estimate that has often been more pungently expressed—"that you feel a little superior to every man who makes you laugh, whether by making faces or verses? Are you aware that you have a pleasant sense of patronizing him . . ." [325]. The comic perspective of life is always quick with this patronizing tendency which can have a rapid descent into contempt and flavour laughter with cynicism. Life is tragic or comic according to the perspective. "Nothing can be funnier", remarks Mr G. K. Chesterton, "properly considered, than the fact that one's own father is a. pigmy if he stands far enough off. Perspective really is the comic element in things" [326]. Our mental perspective does determine whether we shall laugh over folly or failure, or whether we shall cajole or weep or speak in daggers: "all falsehoods, all vices, seen at sufficient distance, seen from the point where our moral sympathies do not interfere, become ludicrous" [327]. Idle laughter, or laughter that loosens a humane grip on life, is always prepared for the vision that persistently looks upon the human drama as a comedy.

But the comic perspective, when discreetly indulged, has its boon and its balm. "If the essence of the comic", continues Emerson, "be the contrast between the idea and the false performance"—and this contains at least enough of the truth to be significant—"there is good reason why we should be affected by the exposure. We have no deeper interest than our integrity, and that we should be made aware, by joke and by stroke, of any lie we entertain" [327]. One great lesson of life is to learn to do without. "The presence of the ideal of right and of truth in all action

227

makes the yawning delinquencies of practice remorseful to the conscience, tragic to the interest, but droll to the intellect " [327]. The spirit of comedy snatches a laughing enlivenment from failure, derives a cheerful gusto from the spectacle of human fussiness in a little corner of the universe, and, when it does not lose its background of essential seriousness, pleasantly converts the frustration of our ideals into genial mirth.

LITERARY REFERENCES

CHAP. I. (1–10)

1 *Iliad*, transl. Lang, Leaf, & Myers, xi, 372–82.
2 *Chron.* II, xxx, 1–10.
3 Bergson, *Laughter*, transl. Brereton & Rothwell, p. 127.
4 Coleridge, *Lectures of* 1818 : *Wit and Humour.*
5 Meredith, in *New Quarterly Magazine*, April 1877 : *An Essay on Comedy.*
6 Saintsbury, *A Short History of English Literature* (1907), p. 332.
7 Freud, *Wit and its Relation to the Unconscious*, transl. Brill, p. 384.
8 Coleridge, *Table Talk* : Aug. 25, 1833.
9 Eastman, *The Sense of Humour*, pp. 7, 151, 167.
10 McDougall, in *Psyche*, 1922, N.S. ii, 4 : *A New Theory of Laughter*, p. 303.

CHAP. II (11–30)

11 Bacon, *Nat. Hist.*, viii, 721.
12 Hobbes, *Human Nature, or the Fundamental Elements of Policy*, ch. 9.
13 Fuller, *Holy and Profane States*, Bk. iii, ch. 2.
14 *Judges*, xvi, 23–5.
15 *Iliad*, transl. Lang, Leaf, & Myers, i, 589–99.
16 Lloyd, in *Fortnightly Review*, 1922, ii : *Humour and Mechanism*, p. 244.
17 *Iliad*, transl. Lang, Leaf, & Myers, ii, 265–78.
18 Plato, *Laws*, transl. Jowett, xi, 935.
19 Plato, *Philebus*, transl. Jowett, 49–50.
20 Plato, *Laws*, transl. Jowett, vii, 816.
21 Plato, *Rep.*, transl. Jowett, x, 606.
22 Plato, *loc. cit.*, iii, 388, 389.
23 Max Beerbohm, *Yet Again : The Humour of the Public.*
24 Eastman, *The Sense of Humour*, p. 127.

LITERARY REFERENCES

[25] Freud, *Wit and its Relation to the Unconscious*, transl. Brill.

[26] St John Lucas, in *Blackwood's Magazine*, 1923 : *Vagabond Impressions*, p. 245.

[27] Kimmins, at *Child Study Society*, Oct. 13th, 1921 : *Springs of Laughter*.

[28] Hobbes, *Human Nature*, ch. 9.

[29] Bergson, *Laughter*, transl. Brereton & Rothwell, p. 198.

[30] McDougall, in *Psyche*, 1922, N.S., ii, 4 : *A New Theory of Laughter*, p. 292.

CHAP. III (31–68)

[31] Washington Irving, *Sketch Book : Christmas Day*.

[32] Quoted from Eastman, *The Sense of Humour*, p. 9.

[33] *The Nation* and *Athenæum*, 1922 : *The Burlesque of Beauty*, p. 49.

[34] Charles Lamb, *Rosamund Gray*.

[35] Cardinall, *The Natives of the Northern Territories of the Gold Coast*, p. 24.

[36] Penjon, in *Revue Philosophique*, 1893, 36 : *Le Rire et la Liberté*.

[37] Hobbes, *Human Nature, or the Fundamental Elements of Policy*, ch. 9.

[38] Bacon, *Nat. Hist.*, viii, 721.

[39] Leigh Hunt, *Wit and Humour : Illust. Essay*.

[40] Darwin, *The Expression of the Emotions*, chs. 8 and 4.

[41] Sully, *Essay on Laughter*.

[42] Milton, *L'Allegro*, l. 32.

[43] Herbert Spencer, in *Macmillan's Magazine*, March 1860 : *The Physiology of Laughter*.

[44] Crile, *The Origin and Nature of the Emotions*, pp. 93–99.

[45] Crile, *loc. cit.*, pp. 90–1. Vide Darwin, *Expression of the Emotions*, ch. 6.

[46] Johnson, *The Idler*, no. 58.

[47] Johnson, *Life of Cowley*.

[48] Conklin, *The Direction of Human Evolution*, p. 18.

[49] Wood Jones, *Aboreal Man*.

[50] Quoted from George Eliot's Essays in *Edin. Rev.*, 1912, 215 : *Laughter*, 390.

[51] Sydney Smith, *Elementary Sketches of Moral Philosophy*, p. 143.

[52] Dasgupta, *A History of Indian Philosophy*, p. 216.

[53] Thackeray, *English Humorists of the Eighteenth Century*, p. 2.

LITERARY REFERENCES

[54] Sydney Smith, *Elementary Sketches of Moral Philosophy*, pp. 143, 138, 136.
[55] Sydney Smith, *loc. cit.*, p. 143.
[56] Bain, *Mental Science*, ch. 7.
[57] Bergson, *Laughter*, transl. Brereton & Rothwell, pp. 135–6.
[58] Bergson, *loc. cit.*, pp. 10–5, 20, 32, 44, 70, 102, 113, 123, 124, 125, 138, 200, 198.
[59] Sydney Smith, *Elementary Sketches of Moral Philosophy*, p. 144.
[60] *Edin. Rev.*, 1912, 215 : *Laughter*, p. 390.
[61] *Edin. Rev., loc. cit.*, p. 401.
[62] Priestley, *Hartley's Theory of the Human Mind*, p. 271.
[63] Sydney Smith, *Elementary Sketches of Moral Philosophy*, p. 149.
[64] Fuller, *Holy and Profane States*, bk. iii, ch. 2.
[65] Oliver Wendell Holmes, *The Autocrat of the Breakfast-Table*, iv.
[66] Frazer, *The Golden Bough*, Pt. 2 : *Taboo*, p. 196.
[67] Plato, *Philebus*, transl. Jowett, 30.
[68] Meredith, in *New Quarterly Magazine*, April 1877 : *An Essay on Comedy*.

CHAP. IV (69–88)

[69] Eastman, *The Sense of Humour*, p. 211.
[70] Bacon, *Nat. Hist.*, viii, 721.
[71] *Loc. cit.*, viii, 721, 766.
[72] Plato, *Philebus*, transl. Jowett, 46.
[73] Eastman, *The Sense of Humour*, pp. 15–6.
[74] Eastman, *loc. cit.*, p. 139.
[75] Eastman, *loc. cit.*, p. 213.
[76] Eastman, *loc. cit.*, pp. 211–22.
[77] Eastman, *loc. cit.*, p. 222.
[78] *Edin. Rev.*, 1912, 225 : *Laughter*, p. 385.
[79] Bacon, *Nat. Hist.*, viii, 721.
[80] Darwin, *The Expression of the Emotions*, ch. 8.
[81] Eastman, *The Sense of Humour*, p. 15.
[82] Crile, *The Origin and Nature of the Emotions*, p. 21.
[83] Bacon, *Nat. Hist.*, viii, 766.
[84] Priestley, *Hartley's Theory of the Human Mind*, p. 273.
[85] Sully, *Essay on Laughter*.
[86] Darwin, *The Expression of the Emotions*, ch. 8.
[87] Crile, *The Origin and Nature of the Emotions*, p. 23.
[88] Crile, *loc. cit.*, p. 22.

LITERARY REFERENCES

CHAP. V (89–114)

[89] Steele, *The Guardian*, xxix, 25.
[90] Carveth Read, *The Origin of Man and of his Superstitions*, p. 60.
[91] Milton, *L'Allegro*, ll. 25–6.
[92] Vide Darwin, *The Expression of the Emotions*, ch. 8.
[93] Erasmus Darwin, *Zoonomia*.
[94] Darwin, *The Expression of the Emotions*, ch. 8.
[95] Darwin, *loc. cit.*
[96] Freud, *Wit and its Relation to the Unconscious*, Transl. Brill.
[97] Eastman, *The Sense of Humour*, p. 5.
[98] Erasmus Darwin, *Zoonomia*.
[99] McDougall, in *Psyche*, 1922, N.S., ii, 4 : *A New Theory of Laughter*, pp. 300–3.
[100] McDougall, *loc. cit.*, p. 295.
[101] Descartes, *The Passions of the Soul*, Art. 125.
[102] McDougall, in *Psyche*, 1922, N.S. ii, 4 : *A New Theory of Laughter*, pp. 295–6.
[103] Thackeray, *English Humorists of the Eighteenth Century*, p. 212.
[104] Eastman, *The Sense of Humour*, p. 7.
[105] McDougall, in *Psyche*, 1922, N.S., ii, 4 : *A New Theory of Laughter*, p. 300.
[106] Bergson, *Mind-Energy*, transl. Carr, p. 23.
[107] Coleridge, *Table Talk*, Aug. 25, 1833.
[108] Coleridge, *Lectures of* 1818 : *Wit and Humour*.
[109] Priestley, *Hartley's Theory of the Human Mind*, p. 273.
[110] Coleridge, *Lectures of* 1818 : *Wit and Humour*.
[111] Lyttelton, in *The Nineteenth Century and After*, 1922, 92 : *The Divine Gift of Humour*, p. 164.
[112] Bergson, *Laughter*, transl. Brereton & Rothwell, pp. 4–5.
[113] Knight, *Colloquia Peripatetica*, p. 118.
[114] Spencer, *Essays*, 2nd Ser. : *The Physiology of Laughter*, p. 111.

CHAP. VI (115–143)

[115] Loeb, *The Organism as a Whole*, p. 281.
[116] Le Bon, *Psychologie des Foules*, 11th edn., 1906, ch. 2.
[117] Sydney Smith, *Elementary Sketches of Moral Philosophy*, p. 151.
[118] De Quincey, *Confessions of an English Opium-Eater*, Pt. 1.
[119] Darwin, *The Expression of the Emotions*, pp. 132–5.

LITERARY REFERENCES

120 Priestley, *Hartley's Theory of the Human Mind*, pp. 271–2.
121 Hobbes, *Human Nature, or the Fundamental Elements of Policy*, ch. 9.
122 Hobbes, *Leviathan*, Pt. 1, vi.
123 Plato, *Theætetus*, transl. Jowett, 190.
124 Emerson, *Letters and Social Aims : The Comic.*
125 Pear, in *Brit. Jl. Psych.*, 1921, 12, ii : *The Intellectual Respectability of Muscular Skill*, p. 163.
126 Jennings, *Behaviour of the Lower Organisms*, Pt. 3.
127 Brewer, *Dictionary of Phrase and Fable*, New Edn., 1895 ; *New English Dictionary.*
128 Höffding, *Outlines of Psychology*, transl. Lowndes, p. 290.
129 Höffding, *loc. cit.*, p. 291.
130 Sully, *The Human Mind*, ii, p. 149.
131 Höffding, *Outlines of Psychology*, transl. Lowndes, p. 292.
132 Bacon, *Nat. Hist.*, viii, 721.
133 Höffding, *Outlines of Psychology*, transl. Lowndes, p. 290.
134 Sully, *The Human Mind*, ii, p. 149.
135 Sully, *loc. cit.*, p. 148.
136 Sully, *loc. cit.*, p. 149.
137 Carveth Read, *The Origin of Man and of his Superstitions*, p. 60.
138 Eastman, *The Sense of Humour*, p. 42.
139 Aristotle, *Poetics*, transl. Bywater, 17.
140 Max Beerbohm, *And Even Now : Laughter.*
141 Bacon, *Nat. Hist.*, viii, 721.
142 Höffding, *Outlines of Psychology*, transl. Lowndes, p. 290.
143 Sully, *The Human Mind*, ii, p. 149.

CHAP. VII (144–164)
144 Sydney Smith, *Elementary Sketches of Moral Philosophy*, p. 114.
145 Meredith, in *New Quart. Mag.*, April, 1877 : *An Essay on Comedy.*
146 *Edin. Rev.*, 1912, 215 : *Laughter*, p. 401.
147 Frazer, *The Golden Bough*, Abridged Edn., p. 44.
148 Aristotle, *Rhetoric*, transl. Welldon, iii, 18.
149 Hazlitt, *Lects. on English Comic Writers : Lect. i.*
150 Hazlitt, *loc. cit.*

LITERARY REFERENCES

[151] Hobbes, *Human Nature, or the Fundamental Elements of Policy*, ch. 9.

[152] Aristotle, *Poetics*, transl. Bywater, 2, 5, 13.

[153] Aristotle, *Rhetoric*, transl. Welldon, ii, 14.

[154] Meredith, in *New Quart. Mag.*, April, 1877 : *An Essay on Comedy.*

[155] Sydney Smith, *Elementary Sketches of Moral Philosophy*, p. 151.

[156] Smith, *loc. cit.*, pp. 148–9.

[157] Smith, *loc. cit.*, p. 140.

[158] Meredith, in *New Quart. Mag.*, April, 1877 : *An Essay on Comedy.*

[159] Sydney Smith, *Elementary Sketches of Moral Philosophy*, p. 148.

[160] Hobbes, *The Answer to the Preface to Gondibert.*

[161] Voltaire, Preface to *L'Enfant Prodigue.*

[162] Max Beerbohm, *And Even Now : Laughter.*

[163] Beerbohm, *loc. cit.*

[164] Flinders Petrie, in *Contemp. Rev.*, Jan. 1921 : *What is Civilization ?*

CHAP. VIII (165–190)

[165] Quintilian,. *Institutes of the Orator*, transl. Patsall, bk. vi, ch. 3.

[166] Aristotle, *Poetics*, transl. Bywater, 5.

[167] Gomperz, *Greek Thinkers*, vol. 4, bk. vi, ch. 25.

[168] Coleridge, *Lects. of* 1818 : *Wit and Humour.*

[169] Aristotle, *Rhetoric*, transl. Welldon, iii, 11 ; i, 7 ; ii, 3.

[170] Bergson, *Laughter*, transl. Brereton & Rothwell, p. 8.

[171] Spencer, *Essays*, 2nd. Ser. : *The Physiology of Laughter*, pp. 113–6.

[172] Höffding, *Outlines of Psychology*, transl. Lowndes, p. 296.

[173] Vide Bain, *Mental and Moral Science*, bk. III, ch. 13.

[174] Aristotle, *Poetics*, transl. Bywater, 2.

[175] Pope, *Dunciad*, bk. 2.

[176] Bain, *Mental and Moral Science*, bk. III, ch. 13.

[177] Edwin Ward, in *Cornhill Mag.*, 1923 : *Round the Easel*, pp. 260–1.

[178] Shakespeare, *Love's Labour's Lost*, V, i, 94–7.

[179] Vide *Edin. Rev.*, 1912, 215 : *Laughter*, p. 384.

[180] Schopenhauer, *The World as Will and Idea.*

[181] Bain, *Mental and Moral Science*, bk. III, ch. 13.

LITERARY REFERENCES

182 Campbell, *The Philosophy of Rhetoric* (1776).
183 *Edin. Rev.*, 1912, 215 : *Laughter*, p. 400.
184 George Eliot, *Essays*, 2nd. edn.; 1884 : *German Wit : Heinrich Heine.*
185 *Edin. Rev.*, 1912, 215 : *Laughter*, p. 384.
186 Bain, *Mental and Moral Science*, bk. III, ch. 13.
187 Sully, *The Human Mind*, ii, p. 151.
188 Höffding, *Outlines of Psychology*, transl. Lowndes, p. 295.
189 Hazlitt, *Lects. on Eng. Comic Writers*, Lect. I.
190 Traill, in *Fortn. Rev.*, 1896, 60 : *The Analytical Humorist*, p. 137.

Chap. IX (191–227)

191 Sydney Smith, *Letter on the Character of Sir James Mackintosh.*
192 Morley, *Aphorisms.*
193 Bacon, *Advancement of Learn.*, bk. I.
194 Bacon, *loc. cit.*, bk. II.
195 Johnson, *The Rambler*, 175.
196 Aristotle, *Poetics*, transl. Bywater, 22.
197 Hobbes, *Leviathan*, ch. 8.
198 Hobbes, *Human Nature, or the Fundamental Elements of Policy*, ch. 9.
199 Hobbes, *Leviathan*, ch. 8.
200 Locke, *Essay*, II, xi, 2.
201 Hazlitt, *Lects. on the Eng. Comic Writers*, Lect. 1.
202 Bacon, *Discourse in Praise of Queen Elizabeth.*
203 Bacon, *Essay of Discourse.*
204 Dryden, *Absalom and Achitophel*, Pt. 1, l. 163.
205 Pope, *An Essay on Criticism*, Pt. ii, l. 97.
206 Raleigh, *Johnson on Shakespeare :* Introd.
207 Johnson, *Life of Cowley.*
208 Burke, *An Essay on the Sublime and Beautiful :* Introd.
209 Reid, *Essays on the Intellectual Powers of Man*, V, iii.
210 Coleridge, *Lects. of* 1818, III : *Wit and Humour ; Miscellaneous Notes on Books and Authors : Fuller ; Lectures on Shakespeare and Milton*, 1811–2, Lect. 6.
211 Sydney Smith, *Elementary Sketches of Moral Philosophy*, Lect. 10.
212 Smith, *loc. cit.*, p. 145.
213 Hazlitt, *Lectures on the Eng. Comic Writers*, Lect. 1.
214 Leigh Hunt, *Wit and Humour :* Illustr. Essay.

LITERARY REFERENCES

[215] George Eliot, in *Westminster Rev.*, 1856 : *German Wit : Heinrich Heine.*
[216] Meredith, in *New Quarterly Mag.*, April, 1877 : *An Essay on Comedy.*
[217] Sully, *The Human Mind*, ii, pp. 148–53.
[218] Bergson, *Laughter*, transl. Brereton & Rothwell, pp. 104–7.
[219] Eastman, *The Sense of Humour*, p. 59.
[220] McDougall, in *Psyche*, 1922, N.S., ii, 4 : *A New Theory of Laughter*, p. 301.
[221] Freud, *Wit and its Relation to the Unconscious*, transl. Brill.
[222] McDougall, *loc. cit.*
[223] Vide Carritt, in *Hibbert Jl.*, 1923, 31 : *A Theory of the Ludicrous*, p. 552.
[224] Addison, *Spectator*, 63.
[225] Freud, *loc. cit.* : *The Tendencies of Wit.*
[226] Traill, in *Fortn. Rev.*, 1896, 60 : *The Analytical Humorist*, pp. 138–9.
[227] Barrow, from Chambers' *Cycl. Eng. Lit.* (1876), i, 391.

CHAP. X (228–253)

[228] Waller, in *Nature*, 1921, 107 : *The Galvanometric Measurement of Human Emotion*, p. 183.
[229] Cannon, *Bodily Changes in Pain, Hunger, Fear, and Rage.*
[230] Bodkin, in *Cornhill Mag.*, 1921 : *Science and Superstition.*
[231] Thorndike, *Animal Intelligence*, pp. 5–9.
[232] Watson, *Psychology from the Standpoint of a Behaviourist*, p. 1.
[233] Quoted by Lilly, in *Fortn. Rev.*, 1896, 59 : *The Theory of the Ludicrous*, p. 736.
[234] Hazlitt, *Lects. on Eng. Comic Writers*, Lect. 1.
[235] Mandeville, *Dialogue between Horatio, Cleomenes, and Fulvia.*
[236] Fabre, *The Hunting Wasps*, transl. de Mattos.
[237] Aristotle, *Rhetoric*, transl. Welldon, i, 11.
[238] Addison, *Spectator*, 249.
[239] Lilly, in *Fortn. Rev.*, 1896, 59 : *The Theory of the Ludicrous*, p. 735.
[240] Darwin, *Descent of Man*, p. 71 ; Romanes, *Animal Intelligence*, p. 444 ; Lloyd Morgan, *Animal Life and Intelligence*, p. 406.

LITERARY REFERENCES

241 Fabre, *The Life of the Caterpillar*, transl. de Mattos, ch. 3.
242 Eastman, *The Sense of Humour*, pp. 189, 209.
243 McDougall, in *Psyche*, 1922, N.S., ii, 4 : *A New Theory of Laughter*, p. 303.
244 Eastman, *loc. cit.*, p. 8.
245 Eastman, *loc. cit.*, pp. 3, 7, 8–11, 14–15, 28, 227–233.
246 Meredith, in *New Quart. Mag.*, April 1877 : *An Essay on Comedy*.
247 McDougall, *Social Psychology*.
248 McDougall, *The Group Mind*, p. 25.
249 McDougall, in *Psyche*, 1922, N.S., ii, 4 : *A New Theory of Laughter*, p. 303.
250 Reid, *Essays on the Intellectual Powers*, vi, 4.
251 Eastman, *The Sense of Humour*, pp. 229–30.
252 Spencer, *Essays*, 2nd Ser. : *The Physiology of Laughter*.
253 Crile, *The Origin and Nature of the Emotions*, p. 99.

CHAP. XI (254–282)

254 Ribot, *Psychologie des Sentiments* (1896), p. 344.
255 Greig, *The Psychology of Laughter and Comedy*, p. 70.
256 Dasgupta, *A History of Indian Philosophy*, i, pp. 432*ff* ; Hume, *The Thirteen Principal Upanishads*, p. 69.
257 Lowell, *Biglow Papers*, 9.
258 Fuller, *Holy and Profane States*, III, 10.
259 Sydney Smith, *Elementary Sketches of Moral Philosophy*, p. 84.
260 Hall & Allin, in *Amer. Jl. Psych.*, 1897, 9 : *The Psychology of Tickling, Laughing, and the Comic*, p. 7.
261 Angell, *Psychology* (1905), ch. 18.
262 Greig, *The Psychology of Laughter and Comedy*, p. 40.
263 Holt, *The Freudian Wish*, pp. 83–87.
264 McDougall, in *Psyche*, 1922, N.S., ii, 4 : *A New Theory of Laughter*, p. 299.
265 Greig, *The Psychology of Laughter and Comedy*, p. 39.
266 Greig, *loc. cit.*, p. 38.
267 Balfour, *Theism and Humanism*.
268 Alexander, *Space, Time, and Deity*, ii, pp. 287–8.
269 Schopenhauer, *The World as Will and Idea*.
270 Sorley, *Moral Values and the Idea of God*, p. 33.
271 Fry, *Vision and Design : An Essay on Aesthetics*.
272 Carveth Read, *The Origin of Man and of his Superstitions*, p. 106.

LITERARY REFERENCES

[273] Marriott, in *Brit. Jl. Psych.*, 1920, 11 : *Mind and Medium in Art*, p. 2.
[274] Jane Harrison, *Ancient Art and Ritual*, 1918, p. 41.
[275] Bullough, in *Brit. Jl. Psych.*, 1912–13, 5 : *Psychical Distance*, p. 87.
[276] Lipps, *Komik und Humor*, p. 44.
[277] Emerson, *Letters and Social Aims : The Comic*.
[278] Dowden, *Shakespeare, his Mind and Art* (1892), pp. 349–50.
[279] Lipps, *Komik und Humor ; Grundlegung der Aesthetik*.
[280] Carritt, in *Hibbert Jl.*, 1923, 31 : *A Theory of the Ludicrous*, p. 552.
[281] Carritt, *loc. cit.*
[282] Carritt, *loc. cit.*, p. 563.

CHAP. XII (283–293)

[283] Max Beerbohm, *Yet Again : The Laughter of the Public*.
[284] Holt, *The Freudian Wish*, p. 17.
[285] Freud, *The Relation of Wit to the Unconscious*, transl. Brill.
[286] Eastman, *The Sense of Humour*, p. 199.
[287] Greig, *The Psychology of Laughter and Comedy*, p. 273.
[288] Freud, *loc. cit.*, p. 384.
[289] Vide Fischer, *Ueber den Witz* (1889).
[290] Vide Lipps, *Komik und Humor* (1898).
[291] Freud, *loc. cit.*
[292] Bliss, in *Amer. Jl. Psych.*, 1915, 26 : *The Origin of Laughter*, pp. 238–40.
[293] Eastman, *The Sense of Humour*, pp. 42, 46.

CHAP. XIII (294–327)

[294] *Punch*, Apr. 27, 1921.
[295] Max Beerbohm, *And Even Now : Laughter*.
[296] Greig, *The Psychology of Laughter and Comedy*, p. 66.
[297] Greig, *loc. cit.*, p. 71.
[298] Havelock Ellis, vide Greig, *loc. cit.*, p. 48.
[299] Robinson, vide Greig, *loc. cit.*, p. 41.
[300] Newbigin, *Brit. Assoc. Pres. Add.*, Sect. E, 1922.
[301] Newbigin, *loc. cit.*
[302] Aristotle, *Rhetoric*, transl. Welldon, iii, 18.
[303] *Iliad*, transl. Lang, Leaf, & Myers, II, 217–222.

LITERARY REFERENCES

[304] Shakespeare, *Richard III*, I, i, 12–37.
[305] Plato, *Republic*, transl. Jowett, iii, 389.
[306] Thackeray, *English Humorists of the Eighteenth Cent.*, p. 212.
[307] Bergson, *Laughter*, transl. Brereton & Rothwell, pp. 23–25.
[308] Aristotle, *Poetics*, transl. Bywater, 5.
[309] Traill, in *Fortn. Rev.*, 1896, 60 : *The Analytical Humorist*, pp. 138–9.
[310] Groos, *Einleitung der Aesthetik*, p. 376.
[311] *Edin. Rev.*, 1912, 215 : *Laughter*, p. 384.
[312] Aristotle, *Rhetoric*, transl. Welldon, II, 4.
[313] Carritt, in *Hibbert Jl.*, 1923, 31 : *A Theory of the Ludicrous*, p. 564.
[314] Lilly, in *Fortn. Rev.*, 1896, 59 : *The Theory of the Ludicrous*, p. 734.
[315] Lilly, *loc. cit.*, p. 733.
[316] Pater, quoted by Lilly, *loc. cit.*, p. 727.
[317] Traill, in *Fortn. Rev.*, 1896, 60 : *The Analytical Humorist*, p. 141.
[318] Traill, *loc. cit.*, p. 143.
[319] Santayana, *Soliloquies in England and Later Soliloquies*, p. 141.
[320] *Edin. Rev.*, 1912, 215 : *Laughter*, p. 388.
[321] Emerson, *Letters and Social Aims : The Comic*.
[322] Fuller, *Holy and Profane States*, Bk. III, 2.
[323] Aristotle, *Nichom. Ethics*, transl. Hatch, bk. IV : *Humour*.
[324] Aristotle, *Poetics*, transl. Bywater, 5.
[325] O. W. Holmes, *Autocrat of Breakfast Table*, 4.
[326] G. K. Chesterton, *William Blake*, p. 16.
[327] Emerson, *Letters and Social Aims : The Comic*.

INDEX

Q